WORKING WITH FAMILIES OF THE POOR

The Guilford Family Therapy Series
Michael P. Nichols, Series Editor

Recent Volumes

Working with Families of the Poor, Second Edition
Patricia Minuchin, Jorge Colapinto, and Salvador Minuchin

Couple Therapy with Gay Men
David E. Greenan and Gil Tunnell

Beyond Technique in Solution-Focused Therapy:
Working with Emotions and the Therapeutic Relationship
Eve Lipchik

Emotionally Focused Couple Therapy with Trauma Survivors:
Strengthening Attachment Bonds
Susan M. Johnson

Narrative Means to Sober Ends: Treating Addiction and Its Aftermath
Jonathan Diamond

Couple Therapy for Infertility
*Ronny Diamond, David Kezur, Mimi Meyers, Constance N. Scharf,
and Margot Weinshel*

Short-Term Couple Therapy
James M. Donovan, Editor

Treating the Tough Adolescent: A Family-Based, Step-by-Step Guide
Scott P. Sells

The Adolescent in Family Therapy: Breaking the Cycle
of Conflict and Control
Joseph A. Micucci

Latino Families in Therapy: A Guide to Multicultural Practice
Celia Jaes Falicov

WORKING WITH FAMILIES OF THE POOR

Second Edition

PATRICIA MINUCHIN
JORGE COLAPINTO
SALVADOR MINUCHIN

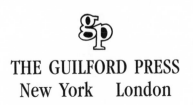

THE GUILFORD PRESS
New York London

© 2007 The Guilford Press
A Division of Guilford Publications, Inc.
72 Spring Street, New York, NY 10012
www.guilford.com

Printed in the United States of America

This book is printed on acid-free paper.

Last digit is print number: 9   8   7   6   5   4   3

Library of Congress Cataloging-in-Publication Data

Minuchin, Patricia.
    Working with families of the poor / Patricia Minuchin, Jorge
Colapinto, Salvador Minuchin. — 2nd ed.
        p. cm. — (The Guilford family therapy series)
    Includes bibliographical references and index.
    ISBN-13: 978-1-59385-347-1 (pbk. : alk. paper)
    ISBN-10: 1-59385-347-5 (pbk. : alk. paper)
    ISBN-13: 978-1-59385-405-8 (hardcover : alk. paper)
    ISBN-10: 1-59385-405-6 (hardcover : alk. paper)
    1. Family social work. 2. Social work with people with social
disabilities. 3. Family psychotherapy. 4. Problem families—Services for.
5. Poor—Services for. I. Colapinto, Jorge. II. Minuchin, Salvador. III.
Title.
HV697.M55 2006
362.5—dc22
                                                            2006034444

About the Authors

Patricia Minuchin, PhD, is Codirector of Family Studies, Inc., and Professor Emerita at Temple University, and is associated with the Minuchin Center for the Family in New York City. Dr. Minuchin has taught at Tufts University and served as Senior Research Associate at Bank Street College of Education. A developmental psychologist, trained in clinical psychology, her publications have focused on the growth and functioning of children in the context of the family, the school, and the conditions created by poverty, foster placements, and family disorganization.

Jorge Colapinto, LPsych, LMFT, is a family therapist and a consultant to human service organizations in the development and implementation of systemic models of service delivery. He has developed training curricula and practice materials for the Administration for Children's Services of New York City and other service agencies. He has been on the faculties of the Philadelphia Child Guidance Clinic, Family Studies, Inc., and the Ackerman Institute for the Family, where he directed the foster care project.

Salvador Minuchin, MD, is Director of Family Studies, Inc., and is associated with the Minuchin Center for the Family. Dr. Minuchin was formerly Director of the Philadelphia Child Guidance Clinic and Professor of Child Psychiatry and Pediatrics at the University of Pennsylvania. A major figure in the field of family therapy, he has published widely on family theory, technique, and practice.

Acknowledgments

This second edition builds on the work described in the first edition, and we continue to be grateful to all those who participated in the programs and experiences reported previously. However, this new edition is focused on the work of the last decade, presenting new material in the areas of substance dependence, foster care, and the mental health of children. We want especially, therefore, to acknowledge the people and the institutions that have been so helpful since the publication of the first edition, facilitating the work and contributing in fundamental ways to our learning and to the results of our efforts.

New and continuing projects have been conducted in three states in the Northeast. The longer-term substance abuse program has been located at Bellevue Hospital in New York; the more recent program has been implemented in collaboration with Daytop New Jersey. James Curtin, Administrator of Daytop New Jersey, initiated the contact with the Minuchin Center for the Family and provided constant support throughout the duration of the program. The newest phase of the foster care project was conducted under the auspices of the Administration for Children's Services, City of New York. We are grateful to Commissioners Nicholas Scoppetta, William Bell, and John Mattingly for their leadership in an area of service that is so complex, difficult, and important. The mental health programs were conducted in collaboration with the Department of Mental Health, Division of Child/Adolescent Services, in Massachusetts. Several administrators in that large system, including Phyllis Hersch, Julia Meehan, Gordon Harper, and Joan Mikula, made our work possible and exciting. We also thank Anne Peretz and her group, in the Massachusetts area, and are grateful to the many people who implemented our programs in the several locations where we have worked. In particular chapters, we have thanked other people by name and hope that we have not inadvertently omitted any members of the working teams or institutional personnel who advanced our efforts and taught us so much.

Our colleagues at the Minuchin Center for the Family have been helpful in many ways. The Center came into being after the publication of the first edition and is now the sponsor for ongoing projects. Active in the area in and around New York, the staff at the Center continues to develop and expand on the ideas and programs that are basic to our approach. We are particularly indebted to David Greenan and Richard Holm, who were the primary consultant/trainers for the substance abuse programs, provided the basic material concerning their work, and are fittingly described as our coauthors for Chapter 5, on substance abuse. In addition, Daniel Minuchin contributed material about training programs for both the substance abuse and mental health chapters.

Finally, we want to thank Series Editor Michael P. Nichols, who was, as always, a knowledgeable and careful reader, and Senior Editor Jim Nageotte at The Guilford Press, who was patient and supportive throughout the process. We also thank the families who are the *raison d'être* for writing this book. In acknowledging the families who appear throughout these pages, we are moved to echo what we observed in the earlier edition: Working with families who are poor and facing multiple crises is a constant reminder of both their difficulties and their strengths. They deserve our compassion, our respect, and our best efforts.

Contents

WORKING WITH FAMILIES OF THE POOR

PART I

Fundamentals of Family-Oriented Thought and Practice

CHAPTER ONE

The New Edition

Elements of Constancy and Change

Why have we written a new edition of this book? Certainly, many aspects of our family orientation and systemic approach remain constant. Yet, as time has gone by, the world has changed and we have changed. Society has become more complex, challenging the helping systems to keep pace in their delivery of services, and we have gained more long-term experience with a variety of problems and service systems. In the process, we have developed a clearer understanding not only of the obstacles to progress, which have long been familiar, but also of the factors that support the work and enable positive changes to endure. In this edition, we describe those forces and suggest procedures to strengthen the likelihood of successful interventions.

This first chapter provides a general orientation to the book. It includes a brief discussion of the changing world and the nature of service systems, an indication of what has been constant in our systemic approach, and a commentary on the search for forces that can enable a new approach to survive. The chapter concludes with a case history illustrating the problems and characteristics of the multicrisis poor, as well as a description of the services assembled to provide help.

THE CHANGING WORLD

With the advent of the 21st century, the world has become more complex and, in some ways, more frightening. We feel more vulnerable than we did, and the poor and needy are the most vulnerable of all; most directly in the paths of hurricanes, economic crises, inadequate health care, and other natural or man-made disasters. If that is the reality, how do current helping systems compare with those of a decade ago? Are they better organized? More compassionate? More effective? Yes, in some places and in some particulars, but, overall, the problems and inadequacies that existed a decade ago are still there.

Current services are often marked by procedures that are fragmented and involve needless duplication, by the efforts of multiple helpers who do not communicate with each other, and by a focus on the individual client without considering the relevance or resources of the family. In a social climate where priorities have shifted and funding for social services has become less available, it's especially important to consider how services for this vulnerable population can be reorganized so that they become more effective and humane. We suggest, in this volume, that a systemic, more family-oriented approach serves this purpose.

Beyond being confronted with the need to deal in better ways with familiar problems, service systems now face issues that stem from increasing diversity in the population and changing social values. Since the first edition of this book was published, the country has seen a significant increase in immigration from diverse corners of the globe, as well as the development of new lifestyles and social beliefs within the culture. Immigration means that recently arrived individuals and their families must cope with the difficulties of acculturation: social isolation, a new language, and the challenge of becoming economically stable, as well as the need to develop patterns of family life that acknowledge the different experiences and needs of older and younger family members. Changing values mean that traditional perspectives coexist with new ways of defining the basics of the social network—in sexual identity, in the definition of family, in the creation and raising of children, and in the very definition of life and death. People finding their way in these new forms must handle conflicts and confusions that have few precedents.

Although these differences were in formation toward the later years of the 20th century, they are now a staple of daily life, social conflict, and legal issues, and present special questions: To whom do children "belong" legally? Which adults should be included in the process, when social services are making decisions about a child, if the family is separated, blended, three-generational, consists of a same-sex couple, or is otherwise complex? What is the appropriate balance between welfare and work, when parents, children, and society must all be served; and who should be making policy that must take into account the different developmental needs of 2-year-olds, 7-year-olds, and 13-year-olds? The challenge to society is profound. We are in need of compassionate and effective services in all areas that affect the health, welfare, and protection of a complex and changing population.

WORKING WITH FAMILIES AND SERVICE SYSTEMS: FUNDAMENTAL PRINCIPLES

Our work has long been guided by two fundamental principles: a *systemic orientation* and an *emphasis on families* as the primary social context for its members. We have carried that perspective through decades of working with people in need and with the systems that serve them. Despite shifts in the population and in the problems that must be dealt with, those principles have always been relevant.

A systemic orientation is both a mode of thinking and a guide for facilitating change. It means that we understand the behavior of people and organizations as functions of connections and interactions, and that when we intervene to facilitate a constructive change, we must take account of the relevant network. From that perspective, it is never enough to isolate individuals as the sole focus of attention. When the services concern or affect children, that point is self-evident, but it also applies to recipients of any age and in any situation. We are better able to plan and implement effective services if we understand the context within which people live; the involvement of others in their problems; and the resources available from immediate family, friends, and extended kin.

A grasp of systemic principles is also essential when we intervene in the policies and procedures of an organization. If we want to create an impact, we need to understand how a particular issue fits into the larger whole, and when the organization is large and complex, we need to accept the fact that the process of change will probably be slow and the effect will generally be partial.

As the reader moves through this book, it will be useful to keep in mind that large organizations, such as the complex enterprise that manages foster care in New York City, and small units, such as the family of a soldier or an unemployed single mother, are all systems. As such, they have similar features. They all contain subsystems and hierarchies of authority; they are marked by boundaries that are sometimes functional and sometimes not; and they must deal with growth and change over time and handle the inevitability of conflicts that may or may not be easily resolved. And, large or small, they must constantly balance the patterns of the whole with the particular needs of their individual members. In the remaining chapters of this first section, we expand on systems, families, and the details of working from a systemic and family-oriented perspective.

WORKING WITH FAMILIES AND SERVICE SYSTEMS: INTERVENTIONS

In the second section of the book, we describe the application of our model in three areas: substance abuse, foster care, and mental health. We have included some projects described in the previous edition, along with material concerning later developments in this work, and have added new projects conducted in recent years.

In presenting this material, the emphasis is on the experience of entering an organization to introduce a new, family-oriented approach to the services they provide. We describe our contact with administrators, the training of institutional staff, and our direct work with families. The material is detailed and concrete; we describe the steps and sequences involved in the intervention process and provide specific examples of how the new approach has been implemented. We also discuss how institutional staff, families, and consultants faced and dealt with the many issues that arise, inevitably, when familiar pathways are disrupted. The aim is to provide ideas and examples that will be useful for people who work in similar circumstances.

THE SEARCH FOR FACILITATING FACTORS

This new edition also discusses our concern with the long-term effects of constructive interventions and with the factors that support such effects. We have accumulated experience over more than two decades, and have been involved with a variety of community organizations. Every chapter in the second section describes interventions in at least two kinds of organizations, covering a broad range: hospitals, residential centers, day and home-based programs, community agencies, and city and statewide systems. Some interventions have been large, some smaller; some have been self-contained, others wide open to pressures from elsewhere. Because of these varied experiences, we have been able to identify a number of factors that sustain the basics of a new approach.

At the end of each chapter, we address the same question: *What enables a new approach to survive?* We answer that question by drawing on the programs described in the chapter, noting the features that have been supportive in that context. Because our understanding has grown by accumulating ideas from the different areas of intervention, we bring the reader through the same experience in reading the successive chapters. We first present the factors that emerged in connection with the substance abuse programs; then we consider the factors that reappeared or were new in the context of foster care, and so on. In the final chapter, we synthesize the material.

The search for facilitating factors is a crucial task for the field at large, both for the institutions that invest in learning about different ways of working and for the teachers who enter an institution as proponents of something new. It's important to structure an intervention so that it creates an immediate impact, but it's equally important to consider what happens when a project has finished and the original proponents leave the scene. Community services function within an ever-changing environment of policies and personnel, and neither the worth of a program nor research about its effects guarantees its survival over time. In our search for relevant factors, therefore, we have considered characteristics of the times, the leaders who make policies and shape services, and the institutions where interventions are mounted, as well as the behavior of the consultants and trainers who bring in new approaches. Not surprisingly, all of these aspects have been relevant.

In coordinating our material in this way, we have been interested primarily in the trajectory of our own interventions and the fruits of our own work. We value the principles of a systemic, family-oriented model, and we want our interventions to survive. It's probable, however, that the factors we have identified are applicable to the survival of any new program introduced into an existing organization.

THE MULTICRISIS POOR: AN ILLUSTRATIVE CASE

Before presenting the principles and skills that are central to our work, we need to bring the problems of poor families to light. We can do this best by describing a particular situation. Readers acquainted with Angie's case from the previous edition can proceed directly to the next chapter, but for new readers, her story is a useful prologue to the remainder of the book.

Angie and Her Family

Angie is at the center of this case, but she's not alone. Her world includes her companion, their two young children, the foster families with whom the children reside, and Angie's parents, siblings, and assorted aunts and uncles. Over the years, Angie and her family have passed through courts, hospitals, shelters, housing programs, drug centers, rehab clinics, day care facilities, and foster care agencies; and they have been attended by lawyers, investigators, doctors, social workers, drug counselors, foster care staff, and therapists. The helpers in this case have been serious about their roles and have wanted a happy ending for some, or all, of the principals. Inevitably, however, they have jostled each other and the family, and often it has been unclear how everyone's work fits together.

Angie, a troubled woman in her early 20s, has had a difficult past. As a child, she was sometimes ignored and sometimes a caretaker for others, and she was abused intermittently and raped more than once. As a young adult, her life has been erratic. She has grappled with drug addiction, maintained an on-and-off relationship with her male companion, and borne children who were removed from her care—a pattern shaped by poverty, poor education, and multiple trauma. Depending on one's focus, Angie can be seen as uncertain, depressed, and irresponsible, or as assertive, realistic, and resilient, or—more accurately—as all of the above.

What would not be accurate is to think of Angie as an isolated individual. In her own view, she is part of a small nuclear family composed of Harlan, her companion, and two young children—Jocelyn, who is 3, and Gail, who is 2. Harlan is the father of both children, and he and Angie clearly consider themselves a couple, although their relationship is volatile.

Harlan suffers from a chronic disease, but he is surprisingly competent in managing his severe handicap. He appears to have no permanent housing and is often vague and unrealistic when he talks, yet he has a strong sense that they are a family. He wants the children to live with Angie, and has an intense interest in Jocelyn, who has inherited his illness. He feels he can help her cope with her condition.

Jocelyn has been in foster care for 2 years. She is unable to walk and appears much younger than her age in speech and intellectual development, but she can do some things for herself and is affable and responsive. She receives rehabilitation services, attends a day care center for handicapped children, and lives with a family trained to deal with her special needs. Jocelyn and the foster family have adapted well to each other, but because Jocelyn lived with her mother until the second child was born, Angie feels that she and Jocelyn have a continuing bond.

Gail, a beautiful, wide-eyed little girl, has been luckier than Jocelyn, since she has not inherited her father's disease, but her life has not been smooth. Angie was drug dependent when Gail was born, and the infant was immediately placed in foster care. The bonding in this foster home is strong. Angie knows she never had a chance to connect with Gail, but she and Harlan both want her returned to live with her mother.

Despite their problems and uncertainties, these people are connected. Harlan and the children are part of Angie's sense of herself and her situation. It's important to keep this in mind as we review the organization of services she has been offered by the community of helpers.

The Community of Helpers

Social organizations have made multiple efforts to provide services for Angie and members of her family. Certainly, the worst disasters have been averted. The city has provided shelter, Jocelyn and Harlan have received medical attention, the children are cared for, and Angie has participated in counseling and substance abuse programs. But these interventions have had complex by-products. The system has sometimes confused Angie so that she becomes less competent, and the family has been fragmented by procedures that solidify the separation and make a viable reunion difficult. If we are to be helpful in such cases, it's necessary to understand the problems created by system interventions, as well as the good intentions and positive effects.

The services provided fall into four areas: professional assistance, the provision of housing, foster care for the children, and a drug rehabilitation program.

Professional Assistance

The number of social service workers involved in Angie's life is overwhelming. It may seem good that so many people have tried to help or wasteful that so much time and money has been poured into one case, but the important point is that the involvement is uncoordinated. Angie has memorized the number on her file that renders her anonymous, and, as the file is handed from one worker to another, she feels impatient with the repetitions. As a result of the turnover at one agency, she says she has dealt with six different workers in a short period of time, and that she's "sick and tired of telling my story to all these people."

Inevitably, perhaps, Angie has learned to work the system, and has been something of an advocate for "us" (the recipients) versus "them" (the system and the staff). Workers have found her difficult at times—"a woman with an attitude." She talks about meetings at a women's shelter where the staff would ask the opinion of the women, and she says impatiently that "you had to do what they want anyway, so why ask?" She doesn't recognize that the staff must work within certain rules, or that they may genuinely want to incorporate group opinion when they can. At the same time, one can understand her sense of frustration and her impression that the system is inefficient and chaotic.

Angie claims that she doesn't trust any of the workers except Mona, whom she considers an exception. Mona is an experienced social worker, whose way of functioning generates both respect and concern in a thoughtful observer; respect because she's an empathic and skillful coordinator, concern because she has taken over much of the executive part of Angie's life. Angie's dependence on the system and its workers is ingrained and has grown deeper with time, even while she feels hemmed in and resentful.

Housing

The urban population of the homeless and/or drug addicted includes a high percentage of women like Angie, whose children have been removed and placed in care. According to both Mona and Angie, the local system has established a Catch-22 policy: "You can't have housing unless you have your children . . . and you can't have your children until you get housing."

Angie has been relatively fortunate. She was contacted by a women's advocacy group and moved into living quarters where children can visit while their mothers wait for official action. Once the children are returned, a family apartment is provided, along with day care for children and counseling for mothers. This new facility has solved some of Angie's problems, but created others. Since male companions are not admitted, there's no provision for Harlan, and an apartment for their nuclear family could not be arranged at this facility.

Foster Care

It would be a distortion to discuss the foster care system as if it had completely failed this family. The children are cared for, and Jocelyn receives the special services required by her physical condition. Nonetheless, the separate services have pulled family members away from each other so that, in the ordinary course of events, they will grow increasingly distant. Jocelyn and Gail are in the care of different foster agencies and do not live with the same foster family. The agencies are geographically distant from each other, have no contact, and it is a logistical problem to arrange family visits. Angie describes the setting for visits organized by protective services as "like a warehouse . . . stuff cluttering up the spaces . . . it's dirty . . . I can't let the girls play on the floor." This is nobody's fault, perhaps, but it is an indication that family contacts have low priority. It's difficult for parents to maintain the visiting schedules, which are usually evaluated as a sign of interest in later court hearings concerning custody.

Even if plans for family reunification go forward, there's little understanding of how complex such a transition would be. There have been many years of separation since the children were placed in foster care, and there has usually been little preparation for the successful management of becoming a family again. Angie is clear about the limitations of the mandatory parenting classes she has attended: How can she answer questions about the way she disciplines her children or what games they play when they don't even live with her? Observing her during an arranged visit, it's clear that she's loving, wants contact, and has some good ideas, but she has few parenting skills for issues that arise in the course of a day with one child, let alone two—one of whom is severely handicapped and requires special care.

There are other matters that have never been addressed, including Harlan's role as a father and the relationship between this family and the foster families that have become so important to the children. In a later section of the book, we discuss a family-oriented approach to foster care, in which procedures would be available for working on such issues.

Drug Rehabilitation

Angie has spent time in a residential drug center as part of the required activity for getting her children back, as well as because of her own desire to become free of drugs. She comments that the program helped her to understand herself and control her habit, but she left long before the allotted duration. "If I stayed up there, I would learn that I could live without Harlan and without the children and be my own person, and take care of *me* . . . but my concern is toward him and the children."

The program presented Angie with a dilemma, but the confusion was not only internal; it was also a function of the mixed messages coming from different agencies. In a meeting that brought together drug counselors and foster care workers, it became clear that each service had its own priorities. The foster care agency was concerned with family relationships and the coordination of Angie's contacts with Jocelyn and Gail. The drug program focused on Angie as an individual, maintaining that she needed to be honest about what she wanted and become strong as an individual before she could deal with other issues.

When a visit with the children upset Angie, the staff of the drug program placed a moratorium on the visits. At that point, Angie faced the contradiction and made a choice, opting for continuing contact with the children. She left the residential program, hoping to remain drug free with the help of counseling—and understandably uneasy about an uncertain future.

In offering this case history, we stop at an arbitrary point. We have wanted only to present a concrete example of the population that comes to the service systems for help and to raise the issues we have addressed in formulating a systemic, family-focused approach to their needs.

—

CHAPTER TWO

The Framework

A Systems Orientation
and a Family-Centered Approach

We suggested, in the previous chapter, that the prevailing forms of service delivery are both inefficient and hard on families. In this chapter, we present the fundamental framework for a different way of working, emphasizing an approach that is more integrated, systemic, and supportive of families. We begin by discussing the basic elements of systems theory; then we describe our concept of families, including both the general features of any family system and the particular realities for multicrisis families in need of services.

THE SYSTEMIC ORIENTATION

We noted earlier that a systems orientation is both a mode of thinking and a guide for facilitating change. We begin, therefore, by considering what it means to be a systems thinker.

We all know what a system is; we talk about social systems, the nervous system, the solar system. The term is familiar, and with a moment's thought, we understand that it has to do with connectedness, with the poetic idea that when you take a flower in your hand, you sense that it is connected to the universe. But a systems perspective highlights something more: the understanding that the parts are related in particular ways. Because of relationships, we can make predictions. Scientists can forecast the moment in which the moon will be positioned between the sun and the earth to produce a lunar eclipse, and they can describe the consequences for the earth and its inhabitants. The parts of a system affect each other, and because these effects repeat themselves, we can study the way they work and predict what will happen.

Systems of different kinds have specific features, but any system is organized and characterized by repetitive patterns. Neither the solar system, the welfare system, nor a family is haphazard in the way it functions. The sun will rise tomorrow and the welfare system will follow particular procedures for supporting dependent children, just as a family will follow organized and predictable patterns of its own.

Connections seem to be understood as a universal truth. When fish begin to die off, we understand readily that certain birds will go hungry unless a functional ratio between these species is reestablished. Yet we are inconsistent in the way we think about people. We celebrate our national figures as if they acted and triumphed alone, and we see the problems and needs of individuals as if they existed in a vacuum, disconnected from their environment and other people. It is a kind of tunnel vision that overrides the basic understanding of connections, and it has major implications for the way we organize the delivery of services. It means that delinquent adolescents and substance-dependent adults are treated in isolation, as if neither their problems nor the solutions were connected to other people.

When we look at how systems are organized, we need to consider a variety of features: the presence of subsystems, the way in which the parts influence each other, and the fact that every system inevitably goes through periods of stability and change. These ideas apply not only to families but also to all social systems, such as hospitals and social service agencies that affect family life. For example, the surgical, outpatient, and social work departments of a hospital are subsystems of the larger institution. Each has a particular function, is related to other departments, and is regulated in its functioning by hospital policies and procedures. Perhaps less obvious is the complex and circular way the parts interact. Maybe the approach of the social workers has broadened the surgeons' way of thinking that "Patient X is a kidney problem." Maybe the surgeons have taught the social workers something about the urgency of emergencies. We're aware that policies tend to travel from the top down, but we pay less attention to the fact that the departments affect hospital policy through the ideas they funnel to administrators and the way they implement or resist directives.

Of course, mutuality doesn't necessarily mean equality. The influence of hospital subsystems on overall policy depends on the flexibility of the system, and within any structure, the power of the different parts is apt to be uneven. In most settings, for instance, the social work department has less overall influence than the surgical division. The point arises again in a family context, particularly if we think about families who are poor and dependent on help from organized institutions. Those families are seldom able to influence the patterns of the systems that serve them, and constructive intervention is often a matter of trying to redress that imbalance.

However they are organized, all systems go through cycles of stability and change. During periods of stability, a system functions through familiar patterns, and, for the most part, repetition is adaptive. Hospitals don't need to reinvent the admission procedure with each new patient, and families don't need to establish new rules for bedtime every day. But all systems that involve living creatures are open-ended. New events occur at intervals, and, as a result, stable patterns are perturbed. One hospital might merge with another and be run thereafter by an HMO. The current procedures would then be challenged. Even if the hospital had been functioning smoothly in the previous circumstances, it would need to reorganize structures and procedures. The staff would go through a transitional period of confusion, searching for patterns that preserve what is valued from the past, while adapting appropriately to the new reality.

Like hospitals, social service agencies are organized systems, and their realities are almost always complex. They're generally embedded within larger social and political structures, subdivided into internal subsystems, and coexistent with other agencies that serve many of the same families. An adoption agency, for example, is embedded in a social–political context that determines legal requirements, the official or unspoken policy on interracial adoptions, the attitude toward gay couples who want to become parents, and the speed with which parental rights are terminated in cases of alleged neglect. These combined factors increase or decrease the number of children eligible for adoption.

Within the agency, work is divided into sections. Particular departments are responsible for different functions, such as locating and evaluating potential adoptive parents, handling legal aspects, or monitoring placement through follow-up visits. Each department has procedures of its own, and the different departments must coordinate their relations with each other and with agencies that work with the same families. Logically, the communication between the department that selects families and the department that monitors placement should be extensive, allowing each to adapt to the realities faced by workers in the other section. An adoption agency should also be in constant communication with services relevant to particular cases, such as the residential center where a child has been living for 2 years before coming up for placement, or the program for children with special needs in the local area where a child is about to be adopted. The connection should be more than a matter of paperwork, especially when a difficult transition, such as adoption, is planned or underway.

Integrating the work of different subsystems and agencies is apt to be time-consuming, but perhaps no more so than handling the negative effects of poor coordination. "Turf" problems between the subsystems of an agency have a corrosive effect, as do communication failures between different agencies. Training is a useful and necessary way to introduce change, but the positive effects are limited if training touches only one corner of a complex system. We've learned, for example, that the ability of line workers to sustain new ideas and procedures depends on the support of their supervisors, as well as on the possibility of influencing agency policies so they can move in the same direction.

A systems orientation is not an academic luxury; it's a necessary tool. Understanding that different agencies are interactive forces within the network encompassing a family is a cornerstone of collaborative work and is essential for handling interventions at cross-purposes. If professionals can accept their connections and find constructive ways of handling their differences, they will increase the efficiency of the system and improve the quality of help offered to their clients.

We move now from this brief description of systems to a more detailed look at the families who are the recipients.

FAMILIES

A family is a special kind of system, with structure, patterns, and properties that organize stability and change. It's also a small human society, whose members have face-to-face contact, emotional ties, and a shared history. We especially need to understand the families served by social agencies. We can approach that understanding best by means of a more general discussion, considering families first as systems and then as small societies.

FAMILIES AS SYSTEMS

Patterns

When we describe families as having a structure, we mean more than a map of who's in the family. We're referring to patterns of interaction that are recurrent and predictable. These patterns reflect the affiliations, tensions, and hierarchies important in human societies, and carry meaning for behavior and relationships.

In most families, there are multiple patterns of alliance, involving people who are emotionally close and mutually supportive. Jerry and Clarissa Brown have been married for more than 20 years. The way they enjoy leisure time together, deal with their family, and handle problems clearly illustrates a stable alliance. But there are other kinds of alliances that are less obvious than theirs. For instance, Grandma and Jenny have a special bond. They spend time together. Grandma is Jenny's confidante and both enjoy the fact that people think they look alike.

Sometimes alliances take a different form. They involve people who are drawn together by an opposition to other family members—and their alliance is more accurately described as a coalition. These coalitions are frequently transient and may be relatively benign. In one family, for instance, the adolescents gang up against their mother whenever she proposes a weekend visit to an unpopular aunt and uncle. In another family, however, the coalition is more stable and less good-humored. The daughters are in alliance against their stepfather, finding a host of ways to oppose him, though they're not close to each other in most other matters.

Patterns that organize the hierarchy of power appear in every family. They define the family pathways for making decisions and controlling the behavior of its members. Patterns of authority are particularly important aspects of family organization. These patterns carry the potential for both harmony and conflict and are subject to challenge as family members grow and change.

Authority patterns that are clear and flexible tend to work well. Clarissa and Jerry Brown have developed a viable process over the years. They defer to each other's authority in particular areas, consider the input of the children when important family decisions are to be made, and have yielded increasing power and autonomy to their children as each one has entered adolescence. Other families, however, have less functional patterns for arriving at decisions and few skills for resolving their differences. Families often come for therapy because their discussions are rigidly organized around winning and losing, and they can't manage to change the patterns that increase family conflict. Authority problems aren't always a matter of rigidity, however. Control may be erratic rather than inflexible, with unfortunate by-products that aren't recognized. In three-generational, single-parent families with young children, for instance, authority may sometimes rest with the mother, at other times with the grandmother, and at still other times with uncles or older sisters—depending on who happens to be around. Messages that are unclear or contradictory confuse the children and interfere with their understanding of acceptable behavior.

Some patterns are ethnic in origin. By and large, families in the Latino community have different patterns for expressing affection, voicing disagreements, and cuddling their young than do their Northern European neighbors. Because South and Central American families have been migrating to North America for some decades, we tend to recognize and accept Latino patterns, but people who have migrated more recently from other parts of the world often seem "foreign" to many Americans, especially if they maintain clear boundaries around their own communities. As a nation, we don't understand the patterns of Middle European, Arabic, or Asian family life very well, but when these families arrive as immigrants without many resources, they are apt to need a variety of services. Aside from economic, medical, and educational needs, many of these people will need help with resolving the issues that divide generations in a new culture: the elders bring values and expectations from the society they have left; the young are exploring the lifestyles of their peers in the streets, in the schools, and through the media. Planning for this reality requires, at the least, an increasing sensitivity to cultural diversity in family patterns, a concentrated effort to broaden the ethnic base of a service staff, and the creation of networks that can provide diverse families with relevant services.

Subsystems

Each family contains a variety of subsystems. Age and gender are among the most obvious examples: Adults have functions and relationships that separate them from their children; males are one unit and females are another; and adolescents form a group with special interests. Within a "blended" family, there are subgroups of "his," "hers," and "theirs." Spoken and unspoken rules govern relationships between the units: The younger children may not disturb the adolescent when the bedroom door is closed; the children will tattle to adults only when beset by injustice; the mother's children will not expect to go on a Saturday outing with their stepfather and his son unless specifically invited; and Grandpa can stand up for a child in trouble with his or her siblings but not when the parents are enforcing discipline.

The concept of *boundaries* is important in relation to subsystems, as it is in relation to the family as a whole. Boundaries are invisible but, like the wind, we know they exist because of the way things move. All of the examples in the previous paragraph refer to boundaries, marking thresholds that should not be crossed, as well as the conditions under which they're more permeable.

The firmness of subsystem boundaries varies with a family's particular style. Thanksgiving dinner at the Smiths brings together three generations, with lots of crowding and a high noise level. That arrangement would make no sense to the Barrys, who put the children at a separate table and call for quiet when the kids act up. In both families, however, there will be developmentally appropriate changes over the family life cycle. The boundaries between adults and children will inevitably grow firmer as the children move toward adolescence. Parents usually intervene if the 5-year-old's teasing brings her little brother to the brink of a tantrum, but when the children become adolescents they're usually expected to fight their own battles; both parents and their children are likely to draw boundaries that provide the adolescents with more privacy. As the parents' generation becomes older, the boundaries may change again, reflecting the needs of the elders and the increasing involvement of their off-spring in their health and well-being.

When family patterns are not working well, it's useful to look separately at the different subsystems. Meeting with just the group of children, for instance, provides a view of family hierarchy and family crosscurrents from the bottom up rather than from the top down. It may also shed light on the repertoire of family members, some of whom may function very differently in different subgroups. Twelve-year-old Mario, for instance, may be a creative and fair-minded leader with his siblings, even though he clams up or is surly when his father is around. That observation provides a useful lead for helping a family explore their own functioning and develop patterns that encompass the needs of particular members.

The Individual

The individual is the smallest unit in the family system—a separate entity but also a piece of the whole. In the framework of a systems approach, it's understood that each person contributes to the formation of family patterns, but it's also evident that personality and behavior are shaped by what the family expects and permits.

This view is more revolutionary than it may sound. It challenges both prevailing theory and the usual organization of social services, which tend to focus on the individual as the appropriate and sufficient unit. We emphasize this point throughout the book, maintaining that an exclusive concern with individual history, dynamics, and treatment is insufficient, and that it's necessary to work with people within the context of their families and their extended network.

If we are to think of individuals as part of a system, we must develop a different view of how self-image is formed and how behavior is governed. Families define their members partly in relation to the qualities and roles of other members. In so doing, they create something of a self-fulfilling prophecy, affecting the self-image and behavior of each individual. Joe is described as shyer than the other children, and he thinks of himself that way. Annie, the oldest girl, is expected to help with the cooking and with the little ones, and she absorbs the role of "parental child" without question—at least until adolescence. Mother is the one who handles contact with the schools and other institutions. The shaping of behavior by the family often involves the recognition of individual qualities, but it may also lock behavior in place, restricting exploration and limiting elements in the concept of self.

From a systems point of view, behavior is explained as a shared responsibility, arising from patterns that trigger and maintain the actions of each individual. It's customary to think that "my child defies me," or that "my partner nags," but these are one-way, linear descriptions. In fact, the child's defiance or the partner's nagging is only half of the equation. The process is *circular* and the behavior is *complementary*, meaning that the behavior is sustained by all the participants. All of them initiate behavior and all of them react; it's not really possible to spot the beginning of the pattern or establish cause and effect. We can say with equal validity that, when Tamika is defiant, her mother yells, Tamika cries, and her mother hits her—or that, when the mother yells at her daughter, Tamika cries, her mother hits her, and Tamika becomes defiant. Their interaction is patterned, and we cannot explain the behavior of one without including the other.

The concept of complementarity has offered a useful, if somewhat startling, way of looking at diagnosis, as well as cause and effect, but it has also raised some cautionary flags. Behavior may reflect a circular pattern, but some behavior is dangerous or morally wrong, exploiting the weakness of some family members and endangering their safety. Feminists have made this point in relation to male violence toward women, and all of society condemns the abuse of children. In such situations, the primary task is to protect victimized individuals and to take an ethical stand, while working with the family to change recurrent patterns that are dangerous or morally unacceptable.

Transitions

All families go through transitional periods. Members grow and change, and events intervene to modify the family's reality. In any change of circumstances, the family, like other systems, faces a period of disorganization. Familiar patterns are no longer appropriate, but new ways of being are not yet available. The family must go through a process of trial and error, searching for some balance between the comfortable patterns that served them in the past and the realistic demands of their new situation. The process, often painful, is marked for a period by uncertainty and tension.

Some transitions are triggered by the normal cycle of development. When a child is born, the helplessness of the infant calls for a new care-taking behavior that changes the relationships among adults within the household. As children grow, there are increasing demands for privacy, autonomy, and responsibility that upset the system and require new patterns. As the middle generation become seniors, problems of aging and frailty require a shift in some functions from the older generation to their adult children. Some transitions, of course, are not developmental at all. They reflect the vicissitudes of modern life and the unexpected events that may happen to any family: divorce, remarriage, unexpected illness, mobilization for war, sudden unemployment, floods or earthquakes, and so on.

Whatever the stimulus, it's important to realize that behavioral difficulties during periods of transition are not necessarily pathological or permanent. They often represent the family's attempts to explore and adapt. Anxiety, depression, and irritability are the affective components of a crisis. Although the behavior may seem disturbed or dysfunctional, a focus on pathology is not helpful; it tends to crystallize the reaction and compound the difficulties.

FAMILIES AS SMALL SOCIETIES

There's something impersonal about discussing the family as a system, probably because it bypasses the feelings and complexities of human interaction. If we look more closely, we can pay attention to the emotional forces that tie people together and pull them apart. People in a family have a special sense of connection with each other: an attachment, a family bond. That's both a perception and a feeling. They know that "we are us," and they care about each other. When we work with families, we know that its members are usually concerned to protect, defend, and support each other—and we draw on this bond to help them change. We know also that tension, conflict, and anger are inevitable, partly because of the ties that bind. As some earlier examples have suggested, a family limits and challenges its members even while it supports them.

The sense of family is expressed by feelings and perceptions, and by the way members describe their history, their attitudes, their style—what some refer to as "the family story": "We're a family that keeps to ourselves; we don't want trouble in this neighborhood," or "We had a hard time moving from the islands, but we're doing OK now," or "We can't ever seem to resolve anything without getting into a battle," or "All the women in our family suffer from depression." There are alternative stories, of course, told by different members, but families usually share some version of who they are and how they function.

The counterpart of family affection is family conflict. All families have disagreements, must negotiate their differences, and must develop ways of handling conflict. It's a question of how effective their methods are: how relevant for resolving issues, how satisfactory for the participants, how well they stay within acceptable boundaries for the expression of anger.

Families sometimes fall apart because they can't find their way through disagreements even though they care for each other. Most families have a signal system, a threshold above which an alarm bell sounds that registers the need for family members to cool down and avoid danger. It matters how early that warning comes, and whether the family has mechanisms for disengagement and crisis control or typically escalates to the point of violence.

FAMILIES IN NEED OF SERVICES: THE MULTICRISIS POOR

Principles of family structure and function are generic, but they have special features when applied to families served and controlled by the courts, the welfare system, and protective services. For one thing, the affection and bonding in these families is often overlooked. We hear that people are so spaced-out on drugs they can't form attachments, that mothers neglect their children and fathers abuse them, and that families are violent and people are isolated. These are all truths for some families but only partial truths, highlighting the most visible aspects of individual and family misery while ignoring the loyalty and affection that family members feel for each other. They generally share a sense of family, no matter how they look to others or how fragmented they have become as a result of interventions that have both helped them and split them apart. Observant foster parents tell us that foster children love their biological mothers and want to be with them, even if they have been hit or neglected. Though this seems an illogical state of affairs, it reflects the deep feeling and emotional ambivalence that accompanies family attachments.

One recurrent and disturbing fact about such families is that they do not write their own stories. Once they enter the institutional network and a case history is opened, society does the editing. When a substance-dependent woman moves through the system and her children are placed in foster care, a folder goes from place to place, transmitting the official version of who she is and which members of her family are considered relevant to her case. A friendlier approach to families elicits their own perspective on who they are, who they care about, and how they see their problems.

Just as connections and affection are not usually recognized, neither are the family structures: the actual membership of the family and the patterns that describe their functioning. Families served by the welfare system often look chaotic; people come and go, and individuals seem cut off. That instability is partly a lifestyle, amid poverty, drugs, and violence, but it's also a by-product of social interventions. Children are taken for placement, members are jailed or hospitalized, services are fragmented. The point is not whether such interventions are sometimes necessary but that they always break up family structures. The interventions are carried out without recognizing the positive emotional ties and effective resources that may have been disrupted as well. When all the children in a family are taken away for placement, the mother's adolescent protector against an abusive boyfriend disappears and the mutually supportive group of siblings is disbanded.

Boundaries are fluid in these families, and workers enter with ease. Often, the family's authority structure, erratic to begin with, disappears. The decisions come from without, and the children learn early on that adults in the family have no power. The worker may unwittingly become part of dysfunctional subsystems, influencing the patterns in a way that is ultimately unhelpful. If the worker supports the adolescent daughter, for instance, allowing her to invoke the power of protective services in battles against her mother, the possibility for the family to manage its own affairs is diminished rather than enhanced.

Violence is a major fact of life for these families, and it takes more than one form. What comes to mind first, because it is the more conventional association, is the violence that occurs within the families themselves. Poverty, impotence, and despair are embedded in the family cycles of this population, often leading to shortcut solutions: drugs, delinquency, impulsive sex, and violence.

When we look inside violent families, we see a derailment of order. The usual fail-safe mechanisms that protect family members and ensure the survival of society don't hold. Any worker who deals with inner-city welfare families faces moments of ugly reality: brutal punishment, incest, abandoned children. As consultants and trainers, we have always been invested in the concept of family preservation and we have supported interventions that keep children in their own homes, but we pay serious attention to the problem of family violence and to the question of how to assess and ensure the safety of family members. The official pendulum that swings through extremes, from removing children to maintaining the family unit to removing the children again, fails to provide a sophisticated solution to this basic issue. The mandates are procedural and global. They are well intentioned but not helpful enough in specific situations. A worker must be able to explore family conflict and to assess the family's potential for positive change before making a decision of this nature. We discuss this important matter further in succeeding chapters.

There is a second form of violence experienced by these families, though we don't usually think of it as such. It comes from intrusion, and from the absolute power of society in exerting control. The rhetoric, and sometimes the reality, is that of protection for the weak, but the intrusion into the family is often disrespectful, damaging ties and dismembering established structures without recognizing that the procedures do violence to the family. Because there is so little recognition that individuals and families are profoundly interconnected, legal structures and social policy set up an adversarial situation, with an associated imbalance between the rights of the family and those of the individual. Procedures are determined through court hearings, where professional advocates present their recommendations and the viewpoint of family members is not directly heard. As a result, the outcomes are usually preordained, following general policies and precedents. The family is the victim, in a sense, of unintended social violence.

Social interventions are often necessary, though less often than they occur and not in the form in which they are generally carried out. If we recognize that the family has structures, attachments, recurrent patterns, and boundaries that have meaning, even if they do not work well, procedures become more family oriented. It's useful to highlight what that implies: *A family-oriented approach means that we begin to look for relevant people in the family network and accept unconventional family shapes. We notice subsystems and the rules that govern family interactions, both those that lead to crises and those that indicate strength. We realize that social interventions create transitions, and that families will go through temporary periods of confusion, anger, and anxiety that should not be treated as typical or permanent. We also become aware that when they are actively intervening, workers are part of the family system. Their role in working with poor families is far more powerful than the role carried by teachers, physicians, or ministers, in relation to more stable and privileged families.* The driving force of a family-oriented approach involves a recognition of these realities and a style of intervention that enables a family to help themselves.

We know that it's difficult for most agencies to adopt and implement a family systems approach, and we have grappled with why that should be so. In this second edition of the book, we are especially interested in the factors that enable an approach of this kind to endure, but it's also important to review the obstacles that stand in the way. We do so, briefly, in the next section, where we discuss three factors that tend to block change: the nature of bureaucracy, the training of professionals, and the attitudes of society.

OBSTACLES TO A FAMILY SYSTEMS APPROACH

The Nature of Bureaucracy

Bureaucracies become top-heavy by accident. They begin by identifying necessary tasks and developing the structures to carry them out. Certainly, the social institutions that serve the poor were created to be helpful: to cure suffering, to protect the weak, and to provide a safety net for society and its members. But the increase in poverty, homelessness, drugs, violence, and the endangerment of children has imposed new demands on protective systems. Ideally, increasing demand would be met by a comprehensive plan to govern the integration of services. In fact, however, the situation has typically given rise to a patchwork of distinct and disconnected elements: shelters, temporary housing, and police action to deal with homelessness; a variety of programs to treat substance abuse; a spectrum of agencies that offer foster care, adoption, residential placement, or clinical therapies for children at risk; and so forth.

The elements of the social service bureaucracy have become specialized turfs, rather than interactive subsystems of an organized structure, and they compete for funds. The level of funding is always inadequate to meet the needs, but an increase in the flow of money would not, in itself, correct the situation. The fundamental problem is that services are not integrated and money is earmarked for specific categories: babies born with positive toxicity or pregnant teenagers or workfare initiatives. Categorical funding labels the territory, points toward certain procedures, and supplies an ideology for preserving artificial boundaries. As a result, agencies and departments vying for financial support shape their language, procedures, and training in accordance with available funding opportunities.

Current policies and procedures focus primarily on the individual. Every case centers on an identified client who has been referred to a particular agency for help with a specific problem. From our perspective, the issue is not that a substance-dependent adult is sent to a drug program or that qualified people are seeking an appropriate foster home for a child; that kind of specialization reflects the competent functioning of the system. The problem is that the customary procedures create a barrier around the individual. There's no provision for the idea that a drug-addicted individual has important connections with other people, or that it's important for the child and birth family to maintain contact through the period of placement.

It's difficult to challenge this individual orientation because the procedures are tied to well-entrenched bureaucratic structures. Budget allotments, caseloads, and insurance reimbursements are based on individual appraisal and treatment. Such arrangements are cumbersome and they don't yield easily. In addition, the emphasis on the individual is taken for granted, not only by the officials who manage the system but by most of the professionals who work within it.

The Training of Professionals

When professional workers ask themselves, "What are we here for?", the answer is usually simple: "To help the patient" (or the abused child, the pregnant teenager, the heroin addict). The focus on the individual is a legacy of professional training that emphasizes individual theory, case material, and therapeutic techniques. Social workers, psychologists, and psychiatrists approach their professional work with a framework of ideas about personality, pathology, and treatment, along with particular skills for dealing with the individual.

Perhaps it's natural to respond to individual qualities and actions, especially if people are in pain. It requires a complex kind of training to respond to the person in context, and to apply healing procedures that go beyond individual distress in order to mobilize the system.

We have yet to reach that point. If anything, advances in scientific knowledge about the brain and the body, the proliferation of medication as the frontline of treatment, and the control of reimbursement by HMOs have reinforced the focus on the individual. In the current climate, that focus begins with intake. Workers are expected to follow prescribed procedures; to gather the required information; and to work toward a definite decision that will move the case to the next step. Though they may enter the system with innovative ideas, workers generally survive by learning how things are done, who's in charge, and what it takes just to keep track of the caseload. It's often assumed that the established procedures are inflexible laws or official mandates: You must fill in the forms this way . . . . You have to arrange visits by following these procedures . . . . This is how you do discharge planning. The professional staff are generally overworked and are apt to view a family orientation as an addition to their jobs rather than a useful approach that's central to the work. They know they're vulnerable, and that if something goes wrong, the bureaucracy will not protect an employee who has not worked according to the rules. The reality of the job doesn't lend itself to time spent searching for families, exploring their strengths, and handling the complexities that multicrisis families present.

If a social service staff can accept the idea that families are a resource, they are on the verge of a more effective approach, but it is only a beginning. They cannot work productively if they do not understand how a system such as the family functions: how the behavior of the individual reflects his or her participation in family patterns, how the actions of courts and agencies reverberate through the family, and how positive changes depend on working with the network within which their client is embedded.

There's an interesting paradox here. Unlike the practitioner in private practice, professionals who work in social agencies are experiential experts on the meaning of an interactive system. In their own working environment, they're aware of hierarchies, rules, coalitions, alliances, subsystems, and conflicts. They're also aware of their particular place in the system. They know that their roles and possibilities are formed and constrained by the way the system works, and that, when they modify or challenge the rules, it has repercussions elsewhere and for other people. It's interesting—and a bit puzzling—that the idea of the family as an interactive system doesn't resonate automatically for staff members. In particular, it should be obvious that the individual doesn't function independently, and that the effects of individual effort are unlikely to be sustained if the relevant system doesn't change. Because that awareness of how systems work may be close to the surface, it may not be so difficult to help workers understand that their clients function within a network.

Social Attitudes toward Families That Are Poor or "Different"

Within social agencies, the effects of the bureaucratic structure and the traditional concentration on individuals are compounded by a view of poor families that is essentially pragmatic and often moralistic. In many settings, the definition of family is narrow. The social work staff must arrive at solutions, and they tend to define family in relation to information that must be funneled to courts or child welfare departments, such as who in a family can supply information about this child's early physical and social history, who might be able to take a neglected child in a kinship foster care arrangement, or where a pregnant adolescent can go with her baby when the infant is born. The staff looks for who might be available to help and who must be ruled out because the record suggests they are destructive in their relationship with the client.

Though definitions are often narrow, judgmental attitudes tend to be broad. Moralistic attitudes toward poor families are submerged but pervasive in the culture. The families are blamed for their substance abuse, homelessness, and economic dependency, and viewed as a burden on society. Separating or ignoring families is partly a reflection of disapproval—accompanied by a missionary spirit when children are seen as the victims. There's a countertrend, of course, which is certainly just as valid. From this different perspective, poor families are viewed as the victims of bad economic times and reactionary policies who react to the hopelessness of their condition with self-destructive and socially unacceptable behavior. In practice, however, criticism and social impatience tend to outweigh compassion, especially when the political pendulum swings in a conservative direction.

Even when families aren't blamed for their poverty or their social behavior, they're often blamed for the plight of the client. They're seen as part of the problem rather than part of the solution. Mara drinks because her boyfriend is abusive, her parents made her feel a failure, and other family members are also drug dependent. Jamal has been neglected by his mother, his grandmother doesn't seem interested, and his uncle said he would take over but never helped him. Jane took up with a boy and got pregnant because the home environment was so bad. And so on.

There's some truth in these judgments, but such a one-sided analysis doesn't acknowledge what the system has squelched, who might be available as a source of strength, or how the family's resources could be tapped to create a more protective and effective context for its individual members.

To this point, we have commented on social attitudes toward the poor, but, as suggested in the first chapter, we also need to consider the attitudes that have greeted increasing ethnic diversity and new lifestyles. Families that have come to this country from unfamiliar backgrounds tend to arouse discomfort and distrust. What are their values and religion? Are they illegal? Are they taking our jobs? Are they a terrorism threat? How can they treat their children that way? When they come into contact with the service systems, they may face not only a lack of understanding, but also policies that compound their problems and workers who carry negative attitudes. To serve these families well, we will need to develop new and thoughtful policy initiatives. We also will need to change the preparation of professional workers so that it includes more emphasis on the diversity of social service clients and on the ways that families from different cultures view the world, form relationships, and function at home and in society.

People who have formed new social units—nontraditional in their attitudes toward gender, toward the definition of family, and toward the creation and rearing of children—will certainly face social barriers, legal problems, and religious criticism from the culture at large. Though people implementing unique lifestyles are generally not poor or in need of help at survival levels, it seems likely that they will be needing services of some kind. We know, for instance, that many people with committed, well thought-out attitudes toward life and relationships find that the raising of children brings on unexpected disagreements, and parents with new and complex lifestyles are probably not an exception. In one unique situation, for instance, four friends who had formed two same-gender partnerships—one of males and one of females—had cooperated in producing a child. The child now lives in the house shared by the two couples, all of whom are her parents, though only two are biologically related to her. The arrangement worked well through the child's earliest years when affection and nurturance were shared and abundant, but as the child has grown, the details of control and discipline have raised disagreements that these four people did not expect, and they have found both the situation and the child's reactions difficult to handle. Such situations, and many we cannot yet imagine, will be brought to professional workers in the future, and the clients may come up against attitudes that are deeply critical and that interfere with the necessary search for constructive ways of helping in unfamiliar situations.

WORKING TOWARD CHANGE

The material of this book is aimed at advancing practical knowledge. We try to provide concrete illustrations of a systems framework and specific examples of interventions that can be helpful in the delivery of services. We know that a staff encouraged to work with families is often uncertain of how to proceed. Workers who aren't accustomed to thinking about family systems lack the skills for effective interventions, and therapists who have worked with system concepts may not know how to apply their skills to agency families. In the remaining chapters of this first section, therefore, we present the material that is most important for training a staff in a family-oriented approach. We discuss the skills necessary for working with families, as well as the details of effective procedures.

It may be useful to note, first, that we've had a particular role in the agencies where we've worked, and that the professional role of the reader may be either analogous or different. As consultants and trainers, we're outsiders, which gives us certain advantages: some freshness of perspective when we look at the agency's structure and way of working, and some freedom from the alliances and tensions that subdivide the insiders. It also brings disadvantages: We must take time to learn how the agency functions, and we miss important subtexts obvious to any member of the staff. Some readers probably share the role we have carried and can read the material for its direct application to what they do. Others may be responsible for training within their own agency and will have a different context for processing the material. The basic points, however, and much of the detail, should make instant sense to any reader who has worked with the complex problems of the multicrisis poor, and should provide some guidelines for people who are planning to move into this field of work.

CHAPTER THREE

Working in the System
Family-Supportive Skills

Social service workers bring two sets of skills to their work: a way of thinking about their clients and a way of functioning to encourage change. If workers are to increase their mastery of interventions that support families, they must develop both a systemic, family-oriented framework and an expanded set of techniques for implementing new ideas. Practical skills are the most direct, involving interaction with clients, but they're not optimally useful or self-sustaining unless accompanied by a mind-set in which the importance of the family and a knowledge of how systems shape behavior are firmly established ideas.

In this chapter, we discuss *conceptual skills* (elements of a mind-set for understanding a family and organizing the information) and *practical skills* (procedures that help families to mobilize and develop their resources). We treat them separately but they're actually linked, and in the following sections it will become clear that they overlap. Examples that concretize the ideas involve some intervention, and interventions are described against the background of our thinking. That is, of course, how skills are implemented in actual practice.

When services are offered, they are necessarily specific, molded to the particular tasks of the setting. In a drug-rehabilitation clinic, for example, the staff must learn to protect or repair client connections with their families, providing necessary supports so that people do not have to choose between taking care of themselves and remaining in contact with others. In an agency concerned with pregnant women, the staff must be aware that the baby has a father who may feel involved in the pregnancy, that it's important to explore connections with family members from whom the mother may be cut off, and that it's vital to fortify her bonding with the infant. Families whose children are in care must be supported during the period of placement, and workers must be skillful in promoting a process of reunification that will be successful for both the child and each family. These are specific issues, but they reflect a general orientation. In that sense, the examples in this chapter apply by analogy to a variety of social services.

CONCEPTUAL SKILLS: THINKING ABOUT FAMILIES

In the previous chapter, families were described as systems and small societies. Now we make those ideas concrete, documenting how we train or supervise a worker to think about the individual as embedded within a context, and to focus on patterns, connections, subsystems, boundaries, and transitions in order to understand a family.

For simplicity's sake, we can say that the conceptual task of a family-oriented approach is twofold: to "think big" and to recognize the organization of the family. Thinking big means going beyond the individual in order to understand important features of a case. It also means a willingness to pause and look around—to push the definition of the relevant system beyond the people who come most readily to mind. Recognizing the organization of the system means an alertness to matters such as the quality of connections among people, the typical patterns of family functioning, the implicit rules that govern interactions, the nature of boundaries, and so forth. The following description of Tracy and her family illustrates this way of thinking.

Thinking about People, Patterns, Rules, and Boundaries

Tracy, a mother of three, gets into frequent fights with her 12-year-old son, Abel, screaming at him and hitting him when he refuses to go to school. A neighbor files a complaint and an agency takes on the case, with mother and son as the identified clients. The staff perspective at this agency is that people are freestanding individuals whose behavior is determined by their psychological makeup. They place the mother in a therapy group so that she can explore her own childhood experiences of abuse, and they send Abel for individual counseling. Later, when Tracy reveals the existence of a live-in boyfriend who is verbally abusive to her, the worker recommends that he also should be seen individually for some sessions. In effect, the staff is treating Tracy's punishment of her son, Abel's school phobia, and the boyfriend's abusive language as separate, unconnected problems.

If the staff perceived behavior in terms of interactions and wanted to understand the prevailing patterns, they would need to think differently, starting with a larger cast of characters. Tracy and Abel are at the center, but also included are Tracy's boyfriend, John, and Abel's two sisters, who live in the same household. They must also think about Tracy's mother, who has considerable influence on Tracy and the children, as well as Tracy's siblings, her godmother, and a close friend. Also relevant are those who are neither family nor friends, but who form part of the network that regulates the life of poor families: a worker from Child Protective Services who has been monitoring the home for 2 years, as well as the truant officer with whom Tracy maintains an antagonistic relationship.

Initially, many of these people will be invisible, or, at least, their relevance and interconnections may not be apparent. Family and friends may not come forth as resources because they are unaccustomed to such a role, or because they're in conflict with the client or each other. And the fact that other professionals shape the family's reality may never occur to the staff. Whether and how these people are included in the work is a separate decision, but knowledge of their existence is important. A large canvas is required for creating a map of the human context. The staff should proceed on the assumption that every family's reality requires a mural rather than a closeup, and that the larger picture must be reconstructed if problems are to be understood and resources mobilized.

To explore relevant patterns, it's useful to begin by spotting central subsystems. The crucial patterns of alliance and antagonism may lie within a particular relationship, in the interaction between subsystems, or both. In Tracy's case, we would know where to look from the nature of the presenting complaint and from the information emerging about John's presence in the household. We know that Tracy and Abel form a problematic subsystem, Tracy and John another. With an educated guess, we also can assume that the triad of

Tracy, John, and Abel occupies a central position in the organization of the family. Alliances and coalitions involving Abel's sisters and Tracy's mother are part of the equation but probably not the point of entry. Experienced workers know they must focus, once they understand the family map, concentrating on the parts of the system that are clearly dysfunctional, or that they know from experience have difficult issues to work out.

In this case, the staff might explore subsystems in which interactions become abusive, noting ways in which Tracy and her son trigger each other, as well as events that bring Tracy and John into conflict. However, they also would pay particular attention to the triad of Tracy, John, and Abel, knowing that boundaries and authority often are unclear when an outsider joins an established unit of parent and children. In this family, the rules of authority were certainly unclear to its members. Tracy and John disagreed about discipline. Abel did not get along with John and felt protective toward his mother, explaining, in part, why he stayed home from school. And Tracy's efforts to control her son escalated to a screaming frenzy, but only when John was present and her mother was not—or when threats from the truant officer became more pressing, Abel more recalcitrant, and John more critical. The members of this network were part of a web of interaction; their individual reactions served as stimuli and responses to the behavior of others.

The particular patterns that emerged in this case are unimportant for our purposes. The point here is that the difficulties of Tracy and her son could only be fully understood in the context of this family's organization. The options for intervention were increased by looking at how different subsystems functioned, and by coming to understand the confusing rules governing family interactions.

Thinking about Transitions

The discussion about Tracy's family provides a useful example of how diagnosis and treatment possibilities change when one thinks systemically. However, an understanding of the family's patterns isn't always sufficient. Families who have just moved into a shelter, or whose children have been taken for placement, or whose teenage daughter has become pregnant, are all in transition; their behavior can best be explained if the staff pays attention to the meaning and impact of changing events.

Megan and her family are in this situation. She is 15 years old and 2 months pregnant. Her mother filed a "Children in Need of Supervision or Services" (CHINS) petition, and Megan was referred to a residential center for pregnant teenagers, where she will live until she goes into labor. There are multiple services available: medical care, schooling, and classes focusing on the special issues of pregnancy, birth, and child development. The staff monitors relationships in the living quarters, encouraging friendships and mediating quarrels, and there are group sessions for the girls. Individual counseling focuses on fears and problems and explores decisions about the future. What's missing is an interest in the family. The staff receives information about why the girl was referred, usually including some commentary about family problems, but lacks the mind-set for exploring family relationships while the girl is at the residence.

Megan is a mildly rebellious adolescent whose excellent grades in school have dropped, and whose close friendship with 16-year-old Jamal has resulted in a pregnancy that frightens her. Though the center of the situation, she is by no means the only one involved. She comes from an intact African American family that participates actively in a strict religious sect. The parents have brought up their five children with firm rules and a tight rein. If the staff were family oriented, they would think it important to explore the prevailing patterns, authority structures, alliances, and tensions that have brought this girl to a residential center. It would soon become clear that the father is a strict disciplinarian; that, though the mother and aunt are close to Megan, they never challenge the father; and that the four younger children obey the family rules. In a family with this structure, the pregnancy is experienced as an unexpected and shocking event, catapulting the family from a coherent, well-organized entity, in which all the members know the rules, to a system in a state of confusion.

Megan's family is in transition, attempting to cope with a disruptive event through familiar patterns that have usually gone unquestioned. The father is in charge, and has handled the situation by ejecting the culprit. The remaining family members go on as before, superficially, but the change is profound and the situation unresolved. There will be a baby, a new member of the family, and Megan will become a parent—ready or not.

The staff needs to consider some basic questions concerning the period of pregnancy and future developments. Will Megan and her baby be permanently banished? Is that what she and the family really want? What are the younger children thinking and how will this affect their adolescence? What about Jamal and his family: Are they interested in the baby? Megan's pregnancy is a transitional period, with fluid properties that will settle eventually into new patterns. Without help, the members of this extended family may settle into their reactions, with boundaries that are too rigid, emotional bonds that aren't honored, and distress that remains unexpressed.

Helping this family will involve practical skills: The worker will have to meet with the family, acknowledging their anger and pain while exploring alternative means for helping Megan and her baby. The first step, however, is conceptual. The staff must understand the traumatic implications of the situation for this family, including the fact that they are in the midst of a profound transition.

Transitions are open-ended. They bring confusion, but also provide opportunities. A worker who thinks creatively is likely to approach a situation like Megan's with the intention of preparing the groundwork for change, and with a long view of the possibilities for reuniting the family. We have worked with families who are angry or distant during the pregnancy but whose availability changes dramatically when the baby is born. The birth of the child is, after all, another major transition, with the appeal of an infant at its center.

If the staff thinks in these terms, they will bring both patience and thoughtful preparation to their work during the pregnancy. In some cases, they may need to reach beyond the immediate family, exploring with the adolescent the resources of her informal network. That network may well include people, such as godmothers, church members, older siblings, or friends, who care about her and will be concerned for the baby. But unless the worker has this mind-set, the development of a support system is likely to be haphazard rather than planful.

As noted in the previous chapter, all families go through transitional periods simply because members enter and leave the family and people grow and change. Most families also face unexpected events of some kind: illness, divorce, relocation, economic reverses, even catastrophic natural disasters. In all those situations, it's essential for workers to understand that families are necessarily in disarray, at such times, and that they can often be helped by tolerating their confusion, exploring the scope of their issues, and helping them to mobilize relevant resources within their own network, as well as through social services.

Preparing for Change

Recognizing family patterns, context, and the impact of transitions allows the staff to approach problems and solutions with a fresh outlook that includes some optimism about mobilizing family strengths. A family always has a broader potential repertoire than appears in its repetitive patterns. Tracy's abusive behavior only partially represents her. Given a different set of circumstances, one might see her sense of responsibility, her tenderness, and her easy humor, as well as her boyfriend's sense of commitment to Tracy's family that lies behind his domineering behavior. Megan's family has strong bonds of loyalty underlying their strictly regulated routine. Immigrant families often have had some success in tackling the unfamiliar, even if they have suffered in the process. These aspects, although temporarily invisible, are part of the latent strength of a family. With help from an agency staff that recognizes their potential, family members may be able to use different parts of themselves in ways that contribute positively to their collective life and individual development.

Recognizing that workers and clients shape each other's behavior is another way of preparing for constructive change. The patterns established in the helping situation may or may not be useful, and even a responsible, well-meaning worker may become part of the problem. In one situation, for instance, the mother of an adolescent daughter came to an agency serving parents of difficult teenagers. She said she was "at her wit's end." Trying to describe how difficult things were between her daughter, Gina, and herself, she mentioned an incident in which she had lost her temper. The worker's antennae went up, almost automatically, and she reacted with concern. She switched from her role as advisor and resource for the mother to a position of advocacy for the girl, forming an alliance that increased tension within the family. The mother was bewildered. She became more defensive with the worker and more helpless in relating to her daughter, while Gina was split between loyalty to her mother and the feeling of power she had acquired through the intervention of the authorities.

In a different situation, however, the staff of a residential center recognized the agency's role in a repetitive negative pattern, and were able to work constructively with the family. In this case, violent confrontations between a 12-year-old and his stepfather routinely landed the boy at the institution. The staff understood that the child's placement provided temporary relief from the chronic tension between the stepfather and the boy's mother and that the situation would continue unless the cycle was broken. They helped the parents negotiate internal differences without involving external sources of control, and they normalized the family's perception of the transitional difficulties that occurred whenever the boy returned home after a period of inpatient therapy.

Preparing to change systems that aren't working well involves ever-expanding circles, including relationships among agencies that serve the same family. Interagency problems crop up surprisingly often in individual cases. When workers make contradictory diagnoses of the family's needs and spend time arguing diverse views, their behavior may mirror the conflicts and unsuccessful coping patterns of family life.

A review of case coordination must always be part of a systems approach. If the agencies are many and their participation is intense, it may be necessary to recognize that "we have met the enemy and they are us." Changing the pattern of agency involvement may require something basically simple, such as reducing the number of agencies in the loop so that coordination is more effective. As a positive by-product, such a move may mean that the family will spend less time traveling to meetings, telling their story over and over, and falling into a pattern of manipulating agency differences to obtain what they want. Whatever the remedies, nothing can change unless a staff is alert to the realities of how things are working, both in the families and in the larger systems that serve them.

PRACTICAL SKILLS: HELPING FAMILIES CHANGE

A broad view of the relevant parties and an understanding of patterns, boundaries, and transitions does not translate automatically into effective service, especially when the primary goal is to engage and empower the family. Many poor families are unaccustomed to taking such an active role. They expect social service agencies to do something *for* them (finding housing or keeping an adolescent off the streets) or *to* them (taking the children away or making surprise home visits). The mother of a boy admitted to a residential center may be glad of the respite, the sibling of a recovering addict may prefer to stay out of her sister's rehabilitation experience, and the parents of a child placed in foster care may be angry at workers in general. Changing those expectations so that the family becomes an active agent in solving its problems requires subtle skills with a paradoxical feature: The staff must learn how to work hard at taking a backseat.

While training agency workers to establish an interactive relationship with families, we emphasize new skills in four areas: gathering information, reframing family assumptions, exploring alternative patterns of interaction, and handling conflict.

Gathering Information

The process of gathering information begins with the first contact. The initial meeting provides an opportunity to convey a respectful interest in how the family sees their situation, even while the worker is learning how the family functions. The basic aim is to make the family feel welcome and involve them immediately in a joint effort. There's a relatively low-key mode for gathering information that consists of listening, observing, and reflecting back an understanding of the family's viewpoint. In the family therapy literature, this is referred to as *joining*, and is the first step toward forming a cooperative unit. More active modes include *mapping* the family structure, or encouraging the *enactment* of typical interactions so the worker can understand how the family handles issues and relationships.

Joining, Listening, and Observing

Families may come to the first session under duress because they have been told by the court or protective services that they must attend meetings at the agency. Or they may come voluntarily, hoping that the agency can somehow fix their troubles. In either case, the worker first must listen to the family's concerns—their own story of what has been happening and why, what they hope for, and what they're afraid of. Their version is just as valid as the official presentation, and sometimes even more so. A busy caseworker may feel impatient with the family's report. It may conflict with the material in the file and thus may seem self-serving or evasive. For the family, however, it is the reality. To listen to their presentation with respectful attention is a skill, and to reflect back an understanding of the difficulties is part of joining, as in the following example:

A young mother whose children were taken away on charges of neglect says: "I don't know what I'm doing here. You people have me running in circles. I don't get any answers."

The worker says: "You're fighting many battles."

The mother continues: "I'm fighting her, him, her . . . (*points at family members and another worker in the room*). I'm only one person."

The worker nods: "You're right. It's too much for one person. How do they fight you?"

The worker acknowledges the mother's point of view and encourages her to continue. Before they have talked much longer, she has gathered information about bureaucratic tangles that aren't part of the official record but are relevant for handling the situation constructively.

When a family begins to describe their reality, the worker must listen with what has sometimes been called the "third ear," picking up on what is said indirectly and registering information obscured in the telling. It's especially important to listen for accomplishments and areas of strength that may have never been openly valued. We know that poor families often present themselves as weaker than they are, especially when they interact with representatives of the system, and that they describe their problems and realities without giving themselves credit for competence. The young mother who has been complaining to the worker says: "They kicked me from the apartment and we ended up in this rat hole without any heat or hot water." The worker asks when that happened and the woman tells her it was a year ago. The worker says, with some force: "You spent one year in that place, with the children!! How did you manage?" She has responded to the part of the story that suggests strength rather than dysfunction, slowing down the narrative to acknowledge the terrible circumstances in the environment—and to highlight the skill that enabled the family to survive.

Listening and observing proceed together. The heritage of psychoanalysis has labeled therapy as the "talking cure," but skillful therapists have always noticed the nonverbal cues of posture, facial expression, and movement. Family therapists have also understood that the family drama takes place, to an extent, right before their eyes.

Observing begins as soon as the family enters the room. The worker must take in patterns and interactions, as well as individual behavior. Of course it matters that the girl looks as if she has been crying, but the worker must scan the group, noticing that her sister looks protective and her mother impatient. How family members seat themselves around the room will also tell a lot about family organization and relationships. Who sits next to whom? Who talks first? Who talks most, and who seems silent, deferential, or uninterested? Which family members support each other and which ones keep their distance? Who relates to the protective service worker who accompanies the family, and who does not?

What about disagreements? As the family members describe their situation, they often tell different stories. It's less important to arrive at "the truth," which is, in any event, always partial, than to discover the family pattern for handling contradictions. Do they interrupt to correct each other, and what happens when they do? Do they argue or insult each other? Does the grandfather ally himself with the children? Do family members compete for the attention and good opinion of the worker? And what of behavior that doesn't fit the family's description? The family may agree, for instance, that all the children ignore the mother's boyfriend, and the worker may accept that as a fact. A look at the videotape, however, reveals what she failed to notice at the time: The youngest boy gravitates repeatedly toward the boyfriend, leaning against his knees while the family and the worker are talking.

By listening to the family and observing them closely, the staff can pick up leads for the aspects they want to reinforce. In the following vignette, the social worker has captured and woven together information that suggests caring, connectedness, and interdependence among family members—even though that behavior is played down in the family's own version:

PAULA: Nobody cared. They knew I was using drugs. They knew I was a prostitute. I don't blame them.

WORKER: But Lisa said she used to go out and look for you.

PAULA: Yeah, that's true. She knew where to find me. But that's it. She's the only one.

WORKER: (to Lisa) What made you go out for her?

LISA: We would get worried. We heard things.

WORKER: We? You and who else?

LISA: My mom. She would hear something . . . the neighbors talking
. . . and she'd tell me, "Go get your sister."

Here the worker has not only underlined the positive concerns of
family members, she has moved from an amorphous "they" to particular people, clarifying the details of who belongs in a map of
Paula's family.

Mapping

A worker who thinks systemically gathers information that provides
a picture of the family. Mapping is a concrete way of recording and
sharing that information. Family scope, connections, functions, and
relationships become more apparent to both workers and clients
when represented graphically.

It's helpful to draw a tentative map of the family even before the
initial meeting. It's a way of carrying a visual image of "family" into
that first encounter. The map would show the members in the primary client's network as the worker understands it from the referral:
their genders and ages, how they are related to the person who has
been referred, and their living arrangements.

The caseworker may know, for instance, that the grandmother has
lodged a complaint stating that the two grandchildren have been
beaten, and that the mother, who denies it, is coming in to see him with
the children. The caseworker is unsure about some facts, however.
Does the grandmother live with the family? Is there a father or boyfriend who hits the children, even if the mother doesn't, and, if so, does
he live with them? Does the mother have siblings, and are they close?
He draws a preliminary map (also called a genogram), which reflects
his tentative knowledge and, perhaps, his questions (see Figure 3.1).

When the caseworker and family meet, it's useful to involve the
family in drawing up their own map. Enlisting their participation can
be matter-of-fact: "Could you just show me here who's in your family? You can draw a circle for the women and a square for the men.
Ask the other people in the family to help you." Inviting family members to place the people and write their names inside a circle pro-
motes a recognition of their mutual belonging, an awareness that
"these are us." It invites them to think about which members are stable, which are transient, and who should be drawn closer together
because of their connection.

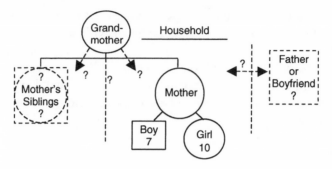

FIGURE 3.1. Family map: Members, boundaries, and subsystems.

The family's construction of their map provides useful information and usually is a pleasurable activity. However, an experienced worker surveys the product with an understanding that the picture may be partial. The first version often fails to include some people—an aunt, or the oldest daughter's godmother—although they participate actively in the life of the family. Questions that show interest contribute to expanding the map: Who else is concerned with Carla's drug problem? (Her godmother? If so, draw her in.) Who might be relieved when she finally joins a program? (Her godmother and aunt? Then, add the aunt as well.) Are there people in the extended family who think she shouldn't keep her new baby? (Her brother and the mother of Carla's boyfriend? Then, add them.) While those procedures are useful, it remains important to be sensitive to reservations on the part of the family. It's early, and, as yet, they don't trust the worker. The larger picture may fill in over time, as the worker and family become a cooperative unit and new people emerge as a result of their joint efforts.

Sometimes family members disagree about who should be included or where they should be placed on the map. Such disagreements are, of course, meaningful. Crystal says, "Daddy needs to be there, too." The worker asks why she thinks he should be there. "Because he's my dad," she says. Her aunt says, "OK. Put him there," but as Crystal writes her father's name inside the circle, her aunt says, "No, he shouldn't be in the circle, because he doesn't live with us, right?"

In some situations, the worker might use mapping to represent more complex aspects of the family's organization. The closeness and distance of family members can be indicated by their placement on the map. Involvement can be indicated by a double line (=) and overinvolvement by a triple line (≡). Conflict can be indicated by wavy lines (≈) and a break in the relationship by broken lines (_\ _). Where useful, symbols can also indicate the difference between clear boundaries (– – –), rigid boundaries (——), and diffuse boundaries (· · · ·).

The Jones family, for instance, consists of mother, stepfather, 16-year-old Lewis, 13-year-old Sheba, and the maternal grandmother. The grandmother doesn't live with them but is interested and available. The father of the children has moved out of the area and has no contact with his former wife or his children. As in many stepfamilies, the mother and her two children form a close subsystem. Lewis is in constant conflict with his stepfather and the mother is protective of her son, coming into conflict with her husband over issues of control. Sheba and her mother have always been especially close.

Figure 3.2 illustrates this situation. There's a clear boundary separating the grandmother from the rest of the family. A rigid boundary, as well as interrupted lines, separates the father from the family, indicating a lack of contact. The placement of the mother and children on the map, as well as the boundary around them, marks this group as a subsystem, and the triple lines between the mother and Sheba suggest overinvolvement. The wavy lines between Lewis and his stepfather, and also between the mother and stepfather, indicate a conflict in these relationships.

Every staff, of course, can develop its own set of symbols, choosing indicators best suited for the families with which they work. A map of this kind helps the staff to think about interactions among family members. Even in its simplest form, mapping gives the staff and the family a shared understanding of the family's scope and membership. It's also a way of normalizing the first contacts between them, moving the meeting away from a persistent focus on problems. As more information emerges, it can be a useful way to record the stability and fluidity of membership, the nature of subsystems, and the family's view of who matters in their lives.

Encouraging Enactments

A map provides a picture of how family members are situated and connected to each other, but family behavior is what offers a handle for useful interventions. An alertness to spontaneous events is an

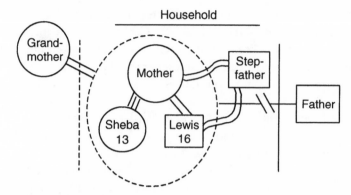

FIGURE 3.2. Family map: Members, boundaries, subsystems, and indicators of the quality of relationships.

important source of information and a skill in itself. However, the role of the worker is not purely that of an observer. To understand family patterns, the worker must encourage the enactment of typical family patterns, which requires a more complex skill.

When family members are interviewed together, they tend to behave typically. Even if they're cautious or suspicious, they handle relationships and events in ways that come naturally, provided they're given space and opportunity to do so. That is a big proviso. Professional workers occupy the central position in an interview and have been trained to take charge—directing questions at particular people, handling tensions and interruptions. It's difficult for people in the helping professions to step out of the action and let it evolve, spotting the useful moment to intervene. If the family members short-circuit their usual patterns by turning to the staff, the most useful procedure in many situations is to channel the interaction back to the family. In the following excerpt, the worker encourages a fuller enactment of family behavior, as it probably would occur in their own home setting.

The caseworker is listening to Miryam's account of the difficulties she is experiencing with her two children, 9-year-old Anthony and 7-year-old Michelle, while they play in the background. Suddenly Anthony pushes Michelle, who begins to cry.

MIRYAM: (*angrily*) Now, what was that?

Both children start to respond at the same time. Miryam ignores them and resumes talking with the worker. The worker, however, sits back in her chair and looks at Miryam and the children alternately. Miryam hesitates, then turns toward Anthony.

MIRYAM: You come here.

ANTHONY: (*to the worker*) She hit me first!

WORKER: I don't know. Tell that to your mother.

Miryam and the children initiate a three-way conversation.

Here the worker is skillfully nonresponsive. She indicates, by posture and by discontinuing her conversation with Miryam, that she will wait for Miryam to handle the situation. Her response to Anthony is direct, indicating that she's unavailable as an ally or judge, and that she regards his mother as the appropriate person to mediate. With these simple but skillful moves, the worker has picked up information about a family pattern: that Miryam may ignore the children's efforts to appeal to her authority, allowing the turmoil to escalate, and that Anthony is quick to enlist other people. As she watches the interaction that she has encouraged, the worker will also see how Miryam handles conflict between the children, and will gather clues about aspects of Miryam's parenting that she can either reinforce or help Miryam to change.

Though the worker's behavior may seem simple enough once it has been pointed out, it is, in fact, not easy for professional workers to hold back. Even experienced therapists are apt to enter too soon and talk too much. Effective enactments empower the family, allowing them to express their usual ways of functioning and to explore new pathways on their own. The worker must be strong enough to take an active leadership role while resisting the tendency to take over.

Reframing Family Assumptions

Constructive intervention is a matter of punctuation, selecting from the emerging information and zeroing in on transactions that are relevant for the worker's task. Part of that task is to help the family members reframe their assumptions about themselves. When a family tells its own story, it's almost always too narrow, and, with multicrisis families in particular, the stories frequently are too negative. Reframing often involves an emphasis on positives, a search for indications of affiliation and affection among family members, and an alertness to suggestions of strength in the way the family copes.

At other times (or simultaneously), the task is a matter of challenging negatives. Challenging the family's rendition of a story should not appear as an aggressive act. Rather, it should offer new options. It may involve helping a child experience how he can make himself understood, though he may have learned to give up before he starts; or helping a boyfriend understand that his opinion counts with his girlfriend, even if he expects to be ignored by her family; or helping a mother realize that she understands her child better than she thinks she does.

In one situation, for instance, Jamie's mother told the worker, "I don't try to get him to listen anymore. . . . The only reason he listened before was [that] I used to hit him, but that's child abuse." The worker tracked the comment: "Are you saying that you don't try to discipline him because the only way you know would be abusive?" The mother says: "Right. I used to, but I don't anymore." The worker had been preparing for this moment and was able to say, "But 5 minutes ago you told him very firmly that he had to put that toy back, and he put it back."

The staff will often need to "catch" a family when they're describing their connections and strengths without realizing what they're doing, or when they're acting in ways that belie their summary of how poorly they function. At that moment, the worker needs to reframe the discussion or the action so that a different aspect comes alive for the family. In talking with Paula about her drug addiction and sexual behavior, the worker caught the moment when Paula described the activities of her sister and mother, and was able to underline the caring and connection in the family. In meeting with Miryam, the worker listened as she talked with her children, and was able to comment later on her competence: "That really calmed things—the way you explained to Anthony how he's supposed to behave here. That was very effective." Through this comment, Miryam's assumption that she can't handle her children comes up for review, introducing a different perspective and planting the seeds for change.

There are many instances when behavior will seem less than acceptable. Parents may seem too sharp with their children, or abdicate their role as authorities or guides. The family's own narrative, which casts the mother as critical, helpless, or out of it, may seem fairly accurate. Nonetheless, the staff must become adept at reframing that behavior in more positive terms—not because it is more true but because it is *equally* true, and because it helps people who feel defeated and self-critical mobilize some other, stronger, part of themselves. When Miryam criticizes Anthony sharply, the worker can say, "You know, I can see you're a very concerned mother, and you have a strong sense of justice." When a mother with three young children watches them banging on the chairs and says in despair that she doesn't know how to stop them, the worker can say, "Yes, it's a problem for you, but you're also very patient with them." That broadens the story of how the family functions, and is a prelude to exploring more effective ways of controlling the children.

It may not seem easy to inject comments of this kind, but it's helpful to remember that people forced to endure very difficult circumstances sometimes exhibit admirable strength and resilience. The multicrisis poor often develop an ability to tolerate frustrating situations that would try any of us, along with useful skills for seeking and using help, a generous and empathic attitude toward other people in similar circumstances, and so forth. With this reality in mind, a worker may find it increasingly easy to recognize commendable elements, and to reframe the meaning of behavior in positive terms.

The effort is important. By shaking up the family's automatic assumptions, the worker creates space to entertain new perspectives. Reframing, however, is part of the process rather than its ultimate goal. An alternative view of family possibilities lays the groundwork for different behavior but usually is an insufficient stimulus for change. It's important to reinforce words and ideas by providing an actual opportunity to explore new patterns of interaction.

Exploring Alternative Patterns of Interaction

Dysfunctional families are partially paralyzed. They're stuck in repetitive patterns that don't work well but that carry some sense of security because they're habitual. The dysfunctional family is often afraid to change, nor do they know how. They need skilled help, which is the job of the staff. Once family patterns are understood and perhaps reframed, the staff must actively intervene to help the family explore new pathways, enabling them to build muscles where there have been none before.

In the systems terms we have used to describe family functioning, one might say that the family needs help to create new boundaries around subsystems and to change the usual rules for communicating. In more down-to-earth language, one might say that family members need different ways of connecting with each other, better ways of expressing their feelings, and a larger, more effective set of skills for resolving conflict.

To overcome the inertia that accompanies habitual behavior, the staff needs to structure interactions that are atypical for the family, asking them to handle the situation and supporting their hesitant new steps. The staff must keep the effort going, highlighting behavior that moves in a more functional direction and redirecting behavior that is sinking back into old patterns. By encouraging explorations, the staff enlists the family as primary actors. The eventual goal is for family members to implement new behavior themselves.

For example, the staff person working with Tracy, John, and Abel asks them to talk with each other about the increasing pressure from the truant officer. How can they work out a way for Abel to get up in the morning and go to school? The grouping itself is new, at least as a problem-solving unit. When John suggests that he could be in charge of waking Abel, Tracy objects, fearing a blowup. The worker then asks John and Abel to discuss the idea while Tracy looks on, creating a new pattern with atypical boundaries. As John and Abel begin to talk, the worker beckons Tracy over to sit near him, physically underlining the invisible boundary around the two males and lending his support to Tracy, who is anxious.

John says he can wake Abel at 7:00, and Abel says not until 7:30—if he isn't already awake by then. Holding Tracy quiet with a gentle gesture, and before John can say that is clearly too late, the worker compliments them on their negotiation, says it's a good compromise, and why not try it. He's basically supporting a new pattern, punctuating the discussion when it shows some progress, and before it runs into trouble and escalates into an argument. These few minutes are only a beginning, but they represent an opening up of new possibilities.

Or, consider the situation of 15-year-old Megan, who is living in the residential center, cut off from her family while awaiting her baby's birth. The staff invites her family to the center to plan for the infant. As Megan breaks down in tears, it is her 14-year-old sister, Saral, who puts an arm around her and offers a tissue. The worker says this is a hard time for all the family, but that she realizes they are respectful of life and probably concerned for the baby. She asks Saral to help Megan talk about how she feels, what she wants, and how she might talk with her parents. The worker goes slowly, knowing that this family doesn't discuss their feelings openly, and that the children don't usually talk together about important matters without parental intervention—especially from the father. When Megan tells her father she would like to come home on weekends and he doesn't answer, the worker asks Megan to "say it a different way so your father can hear what you're trying to tell him." The worker needs to enlist family members to help each other in a difficult situation, reinforcing all efforts to communicate and normalizing the expression of anger, pain, and dependence. Though the exact procedures evolve with the situation, staff intervention to help families explore their own possibilities and solutions is important.

Finally, there is the example of the Silva family, which we can briefly track through the gathering of information, the reframing of the family's assumptions, and the exploration of new patterns.

The worker has received a report of child abuse, stating that Ms. Silva has allegedly hit her 14-year-old daughter, Tina, with a stick. The worker has little other information about the family and his preliminary map includes only these two people. He asks Ms. Silva to come in with Tina. Early in the meeting, they are exploring the reported incident and the following interchange takes place:

WORKER: (to Tina) Do you remember what the stick looked like?

TINA: It was from the broomstick.

WORKER: Where did she hit you?

TINA: Well, she started beating on my leg. My grandmother was telling me, "Run." She said, "Run." My mother was swinging at my face. Then I run to the room, and . . .

WORKER: Wait a minute. Where did your grandmother come from?

TINA: This was in my grandmother's house.

MS. SILVA: That time that I hit her, right. That weekend I went to my mother's house. My mother sent her to the store and she left, and was away for hours, and I hit her.

WORKER: Let me ask you a question. How often did you do that, hitting her with a broomstick?

MS. SILVA: Only that time. Other times I hit her, but not with a broomstick.

WORKER: Well, do you think if that had happened in your home, just with the two of you, you'd still have hit her with a broomstick? Let's say that you are in your home and she takes off without permission.

MS. SILVA: She did do that here.

WORKER: But you didn't hit her with a broomstick.

TINA: She wasn't allowed to. It would be child abuse.

MS. SILVA: No, it's not that I wasn't allowed to. I try to control myself.

WORKER: When you are at home. Do you have broomsticks in your home?

TINA: Of course she does. She can't sweep without a broom.

WORKER: But she never hit you with a broomstick at home.

MS. SILVA: See, but with my mother she knew how to get her way, when my mother sent her to the store.

WORKER: She tricked your mother.

MS. SILVA: Right. Here she could do the same thing. She's done it. But I don't let her get away with it.

WORKER: So maybe the one you wanted to beat with a broom was your mom, for letting your daughter get her way.

TINA: She told my grandmother that if my grandmother didn't walk away she would hit my grandmother. And my grandmother said, "What? That you are going to hit who? I will beat you!"

MS. SILVA: No, it wasn't like that. I told her to move out of the way, because if she didn't she was going to get hit with the stick, not that I was going to hit her with it. My mother didn't want me to hit my daughter.

WORKER: (to Tina) I think you got hit with a broomstick because your mom was trying to teach a lesson to your grandmother.

TINA: And my grandmother would beat her butt.

In this brief interchange, the worker has gathered information and begun to reframe the situation. He has picked up on a passing mention of the grandmother, realizing that the central cast of characters must be expanded. In the subsequent discussion, he reframes the abusive behavior, highlighting the interaction of the mother and grandmother as an important factor.

In planning to explore new patterns, the worker utilizes information he has gathered and considers how the family could most usefully explore new possibilities. The worker has noticed, for instance, that Tina has learned to ally herself with one adult against another. She has been strengthened in challenging her mother's authority, not only by her alliance with her grandmother but also by invoking the power of the authorities in monitoring child abuse. The protection of children from physical harm is an important responsibility of the state, but is not helpful when used as a weapon in the conflict between an adolescent and a parent—especially if the parent's behavior is neither habitual nor severe. In this case, the worker decides to focus on the family triangle and to draw a firm boundary between family members and the authorities. He will encourage an open discussion between mother and grandmother, challenging the coalition between grandmother and Tina in opposition to Ms. Silva, and removing Tina from the inappropriate position of power that increases tension between mother and daughter and leads to physical action.

The worker meets with Ms. Silva, her mother, and Tina. He asks the two adults to discuss their views of how to control Tina. When Tina intrudes to make a comment, the worker stops her: "No, this is something they have to discuss without you." As the discussion develops—or at another meeting, if things go slowly—there will be time to help the mother and/or the grandmother to take over the role of preventing Tina from entering their discussions. That is a new pattern, which must be integrated by the family into their daily life and become self-propelled and automatic. At the same time, the worker and the family need to recognize that Tina is a young adolescent looking for more autonomy. Mother and daughter will need to negotiate some new rules that take into account her changing needs.

In all of these situations, the examples are partial, only suggesting what skills are required. As the work evolves, the staff needs to follow developments, helping the family rehearse new patterns, accept setbacks, and take responsibility for creating its own new and more functional reality.

Handling Conflict

Some of the examples in this chapter involve family conflict, but the question of how to handle conflict is so important that it bears further discussion.

To begin with, there is a theoretical issue about working directly on negative family patterns. Especially for a population that has experienced so much misery and has internalized so much social criticism, it's important to highlight family strengths, reframe negatives, focus on solutions, and empower family members through respect for their viewpoints and support for their efforts. In this chapter, we have focused principally on ways to implement that approach. However, accentuating the positive may be insufficient if a family has not learned to handle their disagreements and their anger. People need mechanisms for managing the tension that is buried, that arises and erupts, or that jeopardizes affection and breaks important connections.

Family disagreements are a part of life. They can be bitter and unyielding in any family, sustained by the unresolved issue of who's "right," by hurt feelings, and by the frustration of efforts that seem to go nowhere, producing statements such as: "I've told him over and over and nothing works", "She doesn't listen; she doesn't understand", or "Nothing gets through unless I hit him." People get stuck in repetitive patterns, hurting each other and unable to see alternatives. The anger may go underground, erupt and escalate, or find its solution in drink or drugs.

What does a worker do? Certainly the staff must assess the degree of danger. They must be concerned to protect the weaker family members and short-circuit incipient tragedy. But there are many stages of family conflict before truly dangerous levels are reached. One definition of empowerment or resilience is that the family has learned to tolerate their differences, and has developed a repertoire for resolving conflict.

Every professional worker knows how useful it is to vent anger. Allowing a client to rail at the system or even at another family member often clears the air, if only because there is a tolerant ear as well as a release of pressure. But conflict goes beyond internal pressure; it is an interactive matter, a failure of communication and resolution between people. The staff cannot tiptoe around that reality if they want to help the family.

Being willing and able to relate to conflict requires a variety of skills. The worker needs to be prepared to stir up disagreement when the family is sidestepping their differences, tolerate conflict when it arises spontaneously, and mediate when conflict is getting out of hand. It is a tall order, perhaps, but the staff doesn't work alone. Members of the family are often effective allies, helping to explore the issues and develop new pathways. The worker initiates and orchestrates the action but may select certain family members to coach, help break silences, or get past the shouting.

For instance, Megan's sister, Saral, who is Megan's ally, manages her father better than Megan does. The worker asks Saral to coach Megan on how she can tell their parents what she wants for the baby and herself. When the silence is broken, the father erupts in anger and the family sits frozen in their chairs. The worker then enters to stir up further discussion: "I understand your pain and your disappointment—and so does Megan—but she's afraid now, and she needs to plan for her baby. Can you and your wife and Megan talk now about what to do?"

The worker is sometimes a traffic cop, keeping some people out, putting others together, providing some with the possibility of venting their anger and others with the experience of resolving an issue before anger takes over. Tina's mother and grandmother need to talk together as adults, expressing their mutual disapproval of the other's way of disciplining Tina, and Tina must be kept out of the discussion. Abel and John need to negotiate the rules for getting up in the morning, while Tracy sits on the sidelines and the worker waits to punctuate the discussion. The worker will intervene at the earliest point of possible agreement, having decided that these family members need to resolve something before their discussion escalates to a conflict—whether or not the plan is optimal.

Tracy and John would need to have their own discussion about how he treats her and what triggers his abusive behavior. When they talk, they will probably shout at each other, an event the worker will need to tolerate, and talk over each other so that neither hears the other—a situation in which the worker will have a role to play. There are various possibilities, and he may use all of them: He may introduce some version of "Hold it! He doesn't hear you. It's too noisy and he's heard that before. Say it in a different way." Tracy would then say something and the worker might say, "Good. Find out if John understood. . . . Ask him." Tracy asks. John shrugs, then says he doesn't mean to talk her down, but he can't stand the way she gets on his case. Tracy is silent. The worker says, "Find out what he means."

The worker is a coach, sometimes part of the discussion and sometimes deliberately on the sidelines. He stirs the pot, sometimes illustrating how a dialogue proceeds when everyone has a say, meaning is explored, and discussion has a longer duration than is usual in this family. It's a new pattern, and it begins to create a new pathway for resolving conflict: fragile, not yet self-sustaining, requiring practice, but potentially significant for the survival of this couple.

The worker has other possibilities, and they are not always verbal. One worker handled situations in which everybody talked at once by calling a halt and holding up a pencil: "This is the talking stick (or 'the magic wand'). Whoever has it can talk; the others listen." Or, in order to make subsystem boundaries concrete, the worker asks the family to change or move their chairs, indicating that certain people will talk about their conflict while other people, who usually intervene when anger rises, will sit at a distance and remain out of the battle. The worker stays out of the discussion but is alert. She may enter to jump-start the discussion again if it comes to an angry halt, or intervene to say to the mother, "This is when your daughter gets frightened and is afraid you'll hit her, so she shouts or runs away. Can you take a minute to listen to her, then you can respond." Or she may bring in a helper from the family to work on different ways of communicating.

The repertoire of skills is broad and the worker uses them flexibly as the contact with the family evolves. At some point, with any family, it will probably be useful to use most of the skills we have described: *to ask people to discuss their disagreements; to keep other family members from smoothing over the situation or taking sides; to introduce other family members in helpful but atypical roles; to mediate—when that seems indicated—by stirring up or slowing down the action; to offer talking sticks or metaphors or even humor as a way of facilitating alternative ways of interacting; and to explore new, more constructive patterns for the resolution of conflict.*

Lurking behind this discussion is the specter of violence, the knowledge that disagreement can escalate to rage, and that rage can express itself in physical aggression. It's the responsibility of the staff to assess the level of violence, and if the decision is made to work with the family, to make the starting point clear: "It's not permissible to hurt the children. There are other ways to do things and we'll explore them, but that's the ground rule. That has to change."

It's not easy to work with family conflict. The staff is often personally uncomfortable, as well as worried. It's a relief to emphasize strength, respect, and support, but agency families—like any others—need ways of moving off their battlegrounds without leaving carnage behind. Or, to soften the image, they need to learn how to avoid severing family connections that are sources of potential support in a difficult world. Megan and her baby need an extended family. Tracy, John, Abel, and Abel's sisters should be able to live together as a family, negotiating their disagreements and their anger. Tina's mother should be able to control her daughter without a broomstick, and Tina should be able to speak up for her rights without pulling in a social worker and calling on the power of the state. In all those situations, conflict can be resolved without harming family members, and without invoking the social interventions that dismember the family.

To work effectively with family conflict, staff members need to factor in a realistic evaluation of their own level of skill at any particular time. They can move on to more difficult situations as they acquire more experience, being sure to maintain the essential staff structures that offer supervision and support during the process. If the workers are to empower families, however, the effort and the risk are necessary.

FAMILIES AND LARGER SYSTEMS: HELPING AT THE JUNCTURE

Many of the problems that beset a family lie at its juncture with larger systems. The multicrisis poor don't manage their contacts with agencies or workers very well. The difficulties are similar to those already existing within the family: confusing pathways of communication, unclear boundaries, weak skills for conflict resolution. The problems are compounded by the fact that the system is skewed, with families in a less powerful position than people in authority. Rebalancing the system often requires procedural changes within the agencies, and we will address the possibilities for facilitating such changes in the next chapter.

To some extent, however, it's possible for staff to help the family relate to service systems more effectively. Staff can do this by

actions and attitudes that empower the family: withholding professional competence, shedding power, respecting and strengthening the
boundaries between the agency and the family. Although such
actions seem mostly a matter of stepping back, they involve some
skill. They require a letting go on the part of professionals who are
trained to take charge, so that people accustomed to a more passive
role can step forward. Knowing when and how to cede power to the
family is a significant skill.

Some opportunities to strengthen family participation occur during ordinary moments of contact with its members. If the worker
isn't alert, they will slip by unnoticed. During an initial interview, for
instance, a teenager recalled being molested by a neighbor as a young
child, and the worker and mother concurred that "she needs to talk
with somebody about that." There was no suggestion that this was
not purely a professional matter, that the mother might be up to the
task, or that other family members might be helpful. In a different
situation, when a young mother was holding her infant during a
scheduled visit and the baby began to cry, the foster mother automatically extended her arms, and the mother promptly returned the baby
to her. Everybody took it for granted. The worker never suggested
that the mother try to soothe him herself, or that the foster mother
advise her about the ways that seem to work best.

In these situations, control and expertise remained with the representatives of the system. Changing the usual pattern would require
some trust that family members will find their way, some skill in handling the moment when they turn again to the expert, and some ability to coach in a way that is simple, useful, and not intrusive. Suggestions by the foster mother about how to soothe the baby, along with
a comment that it doesn't always work, would give the birth mother
some guidance, while protecting the young mother's relationship
with her child and encouraging the growth of competence.

Another way of strengthening the family's role is to search assid-
uously for resources within the family before automatically making a
referral. To do this, the worker must accept that there is a trade-off.
The family is apt to be less knowledgeable and efficient than professional helpers, but they can probably use the mechanisms they work
out themselves in a more sustained way. Maybe a young boy's uncle,
rather than a worker, can coach him on how to stay away from fights
in school. Maybe older siblings can help a teenager with an incipient
drug problem. And maybe the grandparents who have their grandson

in kinship care can negotiate directly with their daughter about the conditions for visitation, rather than automatically relying on rules set by the agency.

To help families regain control over their lives, the staff must rein in the impulse to refer every situation to an expert, and they must monitor their own controlling behavior, asking themselves in each instance whether an intervention is really necessary. Whatever the answer, there should be a pause between impulse and action; control should be a function of necessity rather than of role.

Sometimes, of course, a controlling stance is unavoidable. If that happens, the worker must find a way to keep the issue from dominating the relationship. When Jane missed her appointment for a urine test at the clinic, for instance, the worker was required by law to notify the agency. At the next session with Jane and Jerry, her boyfriend, Jane was angry.

JANE: I don't feel like having a session today.

WORKER: How come?

JANE: I'm pissed. I miss one f____ test and you report me.

WORKER: Well, the rules are that if you miss a test, I have to report it and I did, but I wrote down your explanation as well. I'm glad you came in, though. I know you're angry at the agency these days and I think you might try to find out from Jerry how he thinks you should handle that.

In general, an effective worker wants to strengthen the boundary between family and agencies, stepping out of the action, withholding expertise, and asking family members to talk together about their issues—even those concerning problems in dealing with agencies. In the following interchange, which involves parents whose children have been taken into care, the worker wants the parents to develop a sense that they're a team, that they probably have useful ideas, and that together they may have some power. The couple begins with the assumption that all the decisions lie outside of them.

WORKER: Have you talked with your husband about what you need to do to get your children back?

MOTHER: He's not the one who took them away. It's the people who took them away who's got to give me some answers. We can't do anything until we get some answers.

WORKER: Who have you been talking to?

MOTHER: This woman, McSomething, at protective services.

WORKER: (*to father*) And you?

FATHER: Nobody. I don't talk to those people. I tell her it's no use.

WORKER: I think you need to work as a team. Why don't you talk together now about how to deal with this.

As indicated earlier, the problems that lie at the juncture between families and larger systems cannot be fully handled by agency workers, even those who are skillful. Progress often depends on procedural changes in how an agency functions, and on the coordination of services among the various agencies that serve the same families. We will discuss procedural matters in the next chapter, and we will continue to illustrate the application of skills throughout the remainder of the book.

A SUMMARY OF SKILLS

Because the skills described in this chapter are so basic in working effectively with families, we close the chapter by summarizing and rephrasing its main points.

Workers must first *think* about families (Points 1–5), then must exercise *practical skills* to help families change (Points 6–10):

1. Families are social systems. They organize their members toward certain ways of thinking about themselves and interacting with each other. The behavior of family members becomes constrained over time by family rules, boundaries, and expectations. What the staff sees when they meet a family is predictable behavior that defines "the way things are" in the family.

2. The typical behavior of family members may be preferred, but alternative patterns are available—even if seldom used. This fact encourages a hopeful view of possibilities, providing incentive for exploring the family's repertoire. Assessment of a family should always include the invisible roster of strengths and resources.

3. Individuals are separate entities, but are also part of a web of family relationships. Staff members are often presented with an identified client whose symptoms or behavior are defined as the problem. They can accept the presenting complaint as valid, but must be aware that control of the symptom lies in the interaction between family members and the client.

4. Families move through transitional periods, in which the demands of new circumstances require a change in family patterns. The family may respond by adapting and evolving, but families sometimes get stuck, maintaining patterns that are habitual but not adaptive. Symptoms or disruptive behavior in one family member may reflect the family's distress. The problems are potentially transitory, and the function of the staff is to help the family through a period of disorganization.

5. When they intervene, workers become part of the family system, and are likely to be pulled toward accepting the family's view of who they are and how they should be helped. The staff should understand that the pull of the system narrows their view of the family. It's important, even if difficult, to think about the family in a different way and to highlight their capacity for expansion.

6. The staff's first efforts to help families change should explore how they define their problems, questioning and expanding what the family has taken for granted. The skills for gathering information and exploring possibilities include listening, observing, mapping, reframing, and helping families explore agreements and disagreements through spontaneous and guided enactments.

7. Workers are the catalysts of change. They help the family recognize dysfunctional patterns and explore the possibility of relating in different ways. Family members are encouraged to connect, whenever alienated, and to explore constructive approaches to conflict.

8. The staff empowers families by focusing on family strengths, but they must also work with conflict. If conflicts aren't resolved, they may alienate family members from each other or erupt into violence. Workers should explore this area, listening for disagreements, helping the family to handle conflict safely, and exploring new ways of relating under stress.

9. Intervention is most effective if the staff can restrain their expertise, using their skills to encourage family members to see each other as a resource and to mobilize help from within their own network. That may involve a new role for workers, requiring a less cen-

tral position than is customary and a less active effort to solve the family's problems for them.

10. The staff should consider the extended family as its own primary resource, expanding their initial view of who might be available to help. A request for additional professional services may not be necessary and should be considered carefully. When many agencies are providing a family with multiple services, it's important to evaluate the balance between help and confusion. One of the most useful interventions on behalf of a family may be to induce organizational changes, so that services become more collaborative, family-friendly, and effective.

CHAPTER FOUR

Changing the System
Family-Supportive Procedures

The implementation of a family approach depends on the skills of professional workers, and the success of their efforts depends in turn on the support of their agencies: in effect, it's a circle of mutual dependence. Agency support is partly a matter of attitude, but it's also a matter of structure, in which the details of policy and procedure allow the staff to exercise a repertoire of family-oriented skills. That situation is not easily come by. It's often necessary to review established procedures, looking for details that obstruct or facilitate a family approach, and modifying procedures so they provide a supportive context.

From our perspective, procedures such as intake, assessment, planning, and service are part of one continuing process. If they aren't consistently organized to include the family from the beginning, it becomes increasingly difficult to do so at a later stage. Consider the following situations:

Angela, a depressed mother of four with a history of sporadic drinking, lives with her children in a temporary shelter for homeless families. When she gets into trouble for curfew violations, the shelter workers invite her husband, who is staying with his mother, to a meeting. He gently scolds Angela for her misbehavior while also praising the progress she has made in battling her drinking problem. Angela responds like a contrite child, and that same night she violates curfew once again.

James, an 11-year-old, is living at a residential center because of violent behavior at school and at home. He has just completed 3 months of residential treatment, and, according to the staff, is ready to participate in family therapy sessions to prepare for his discharge. During the first session, James and his mother engage in a heated argument and the stepfather storms out of the room, swearing that either James will have to leave the family or he will.

Laura's newborn, Wanda, is placed in foster care so that her mother can attend a residential drug-treatment program. After 6 months, during which Laura sees her daughter once every other week, the child welfare and foster care agencies decide that mother and daughter are ready to be reunited. The foster care staff increases the frequency of visits and complements them with weekly family sessions for Laura, Wanda, and Laura's new boyfriend. However, the couple seems uninterested, misses appointments, and hints that Wanda might need to stay longer in foster care to give her mother time to adjust.

In these situations, the workers were handling crises and transitions by trying to apply their newly acquired skills for working with families. When Angela broke curfew, the workers reached out to the man who was presumably important in her life, and when James and Laura were deemed ready, the staff began to reconnect parents and children. But, in each case, it was too late. None of the services had created an involvement with the family before that moment. James and Laura had been purposely separated from their families so that their individual problems could be treated without interference from the issues of daily life, and Angela's husband had never been contacted by the staff, though he had come to the shelter for occasional visits.

If agency procedures had been different from the start, events might have taken a different course. What if Angela's husband had been encouraged from the beginning to remain involved with his family? Angela might not have violated curfew. Or, if it had become clear that he was not the best resource for Angela, the staff could have explored other avenues of support. What about James and

Laura? If family sessions had started earlier, James's family might have handled the transitional issues more constructively when the staff thought the child was ready to return to the family. In a similar manner, the relationship between Laura and her baby might have been more solid if they had had frequent contact during those first 6 months after Wanda's birth.

When agency procedures are codified into a particular routine for intake and service that does not include families, the workers follow the established pattern. Angela's application for a place in the shelter was treated as if she had been a single parent; her husband was not included. James was treated at the residential center while his family waited outside, both literally and symbolically. And Wanda was placed in some kind of layaway while her mother was sent to recover from drugs. The procedures began with the individual as the focus of concern, leaving little room for the practice of family-oriented skills, and making it unlikely that family members could respond helpfully at a point of crisis or transition.

The first contact with the agency is crucial; it establishes the tone of everything that follows. In the second part of the book, which describes the introduction of family-oriented programs into a variety of particular settings, the effort to encourage an intake process that includes the family is placed in context, and examples of the obstacles that are frequently faced and the conditions that support a positive change are provided. In the section below, however, we present material that is generally applicable in a variety of situations, offering a detailed and sequential discussion of how to proceed with a family-supportive approach at the point of intake.

INTAKE: FORMING A PARTNERSHIP WITH THE FAMILY

When a new case comes to an agency, there's a flurry of urgent work to be done. Intake is a period for gathering information, filling out forms, and making decisions that will connect the client to a new setting and to the professionals who will provide services. Not necessarily a crisis, but not a time for dallying either. Agency workers feel the pressure: They're aware that the relay race started farther back and higher up, that they must carry it forward, and that they're responsible to the larger systems that made the referral and expect accountability in return. The pressure and official forms often dictate the

intake process, leading to a focus on the diagnosis of individual dysfunction (e.g., "drug addiction," "depression," "acting out," "poor
parenting skills") and on the familiar categories of information that
usually fill the official record (e.g., individual history, cognitive and
emotional status, diagnosis, motivation, prognosis).

Within these parameters, the inclusion of the client's family at
the point of intake may seem complicated, troublesome, and perhaps
unnecessary. Even if the agency expects to work with the family—as
in the examples cited earlier—it's often the policy or assumption that
such work will come later, when the client is deemed ready. First it's
necessary to deal with the presenting problem of the identified client.
Procedures and planning must move along established pathways.

If an agency wishes to create an active partnership with families,
it must usually arrange a radical revision of the customary procedures, beginning with a concerted effort to maximize the involvement of the family in the intake process. The family should emerge
from the first contact with a sense that the staff is respectful, supportive, and concerned with understanding the family's perspective.
The staff should make it clear that the agency will regard them as
partners in the development of solutions, and that their continuing
involvement in treatment is essential.

Given the critical importance of this initial phase, we will look at
the procedures of intake in detail, considering who to invite, what to
cover, and how to assess and relate to the family. We take these procedures step-by-step, indicating the sequence of events and the decisions to be made. This process is basically in the hands of the workers who receive the family, but the staff must have agency support at
several levels, ranging from flexibility in timing to new intake forms
that guide the interview toward the inclusion of family matters.

Whom to Invite

The question of whom to invite harks back to a family-oriented
mind-set and to the mandate "think big." Here are the identified clients: Angela, James, Laura. Who are the important people in the life
space of each? In the previous chapter, we traced that through for
Tracy and Abel, knowing we must include John, Tracy's mother, and
Abel's sisters, at the very least. Likewise, we have also populated the
personal world of the three people introduced in this chapter by noting the central role of husbands, boyfriends, parents, and children.

How does the staff arrive at an understanding of the relevant people, and how do they decide whom to invite to the very first meeting?

As suggested earlier, it's useful to make a map from the known facts on the referral sheet, but it's also important to consider the probabilities. Teenagers usually have a parent somewhere out there, even if they come in alone, and they may have concerned aunts, grandparents, siblings, or close friends. Children often have more than one adult involved in their lives, even if the mother is central and is a reliable source for all the usual questions. Workers would do well to have an automatic checklist in their heads of who might be involved, including not only immediate kin and members of the household but also stable or transitory companions, siblings who don't live at home, foster family members, church and school personnel, and a variety of workers who may provide continuity from the past and facilitate an assessment of current realities and resources.

If all of these people were included at the outset, the stage would be crowded and the process possibly unproductive. It's important, however, to consider who might be relevant and then make choices from a broad array of people. The fragmentation created by the system, or by the erratic life history of the client, should not limit the caseworker who sets up the initial meetings.

What actually happens at intake is controlled by the worker's judgment and by practical realities. Sometimes the very first contact is created by happenstance. Angela and her children may have been brought to the shelter on a bitter winter evening by the police: no husband in sight, and no grandmother, church member, or worker from the housing unit. James may have been brought to the residential center by his mother after a violent tantrum at school and an emergency referral by the school counselor: no stepfather present, and no siblings, no representative of the school. Of course, the process must begin at that point, with admission and a few essential papers. But conversation is crucial, and should include the assurance that staff and family will explore this situation together as soon as possible. It's at this first encounter that the worker establishes the necessity of family participation, mapping out with Angela or James and his mother who is important in the larger picture and who should be present at the next meeting.

Through this first contact, or even from the official records, it may be clear who should participate in the intake, but they don't necessarily gather together with ease. Some family members are reluctant to attend because they're at odds with each other, or because they fear being blamed. Parents whose children have been forcibly removed may be resentful or depressed, and don't see any point in making contact with the foster care agency. James's stepfather may blame his wife for the boy's behavior and decide it's best if he keeps his distance. Laura may be reluctant to involve her family out of anger or fear or pride. And professional workers from other agencies may not want to attend a meeting after moving a client off their caseload; they have too much to do and are unfamiliar with this procedure.

The staff must meet these situations with a clear message about the necessity of participation that can be heard by the clients and that fits the possibilities of the setting. For example, a residential center in Sweden brings the family in to live for a week with the child, and a hospital director in the United States has redesigned space in the children's ward so that the family can spend the first day and night together. Those are bold measures and not always possible, but there are many other ways to convey the message and accommodate the participants. A foster care agency may need to make an extra effort to contact and involve the child's biological family at the point of placement. The invitation to this family should carry the message: "We need you. Without your help, we will have more difficulty making this placement work for your child."

Sometimes a matter-of-fact approach is useful. In a drug rehabilitation clinic, for instance, it's possible to make family participation a condition for admission. As the director of one clinic put it, "We can take the position, as we do with urine samples, that the family intake is not negotiable." Similarly, when a child comes in to a ward or residential center, the staff can convey the idea that of course the father will be involved—even if the mother is the parent who usually deals with outside institutions. As fathers, working mothers, siblings, and other professionals may find it difficult to leave work or school to attend the intake, the agency will need to accommodate them, offering flexible scheduling that includes evening or weekend hours.

The ideal of broad participation must be tempered by the judgment of the staff, as well as by practical considerations. When family therapists first meet with a family, they usually want to see the array of relevant people, but subsequent meetings are arranged with subsets and combinations, depending on what they deem useful. The same kind of appraisal is required in the agency setting, although the context and complexity of the families set up a different challenge. The main purpose is to establish connections and not overwhelm the primary client or the family. For that reason, it may be unproductive to start the intake with everybody who appears relevant, though it's always important to expand the cast beyond traditional expectations.

The very first contact provides some idea of who the client sees as allies or adversaries, and what the sore spots are. It would have been clear from the first conversation with James and his mother that the mother and stepfather disagreed about how to handle him, and that the godmother, who lives nearby, supported the mother and was an important force. Armed with that information, the worker might have decided to invite the two parents first, because their conflicting viewpoints are a central part of the situation, adding the godmother, 14-year-old sister, and school counselor in subsequent meetings. Angela's husband would have been included immediately, to acknowledge his role and assess their relationship, while later sessions might have included his mother, the housing worker, and Angela's sister, or a friend from Angela's church. If Laura had indicated that her mother didn't help out because she was very angry, the worker might have decided not to increase the tension of the first meeting by including her. Rather, she might have assembled Laura and her boyfriend for the first extended contact, moving on in subsequent meetings to include the baby, the foster mother, the child care worker, and perhaps Laura's mother as a potential resource.

These decisions involve clinical judgments, and must include multiple factors. Newly trained workers must take account of their own fledgling skills and their level of comfort in handling conflict. Any intake worker must expand the cast of characters beyond the individual, but workers finding their way in the face of family resistance may need to gauge the balance of conflict and support in the family system so that those invited to the meeting will not bring an unmanageable level of family tension. In this evaluation, the preference of the primary client can be useful. In one clinic, the staff offers reluctant clients the option of inviting two family members of their choice to the session. They assume that people chosen in this way will offer a broader perspective and will also support the client through the early stages of admission and participation.

Intake may actually take place over several meetings, during which relevant people are invited sequentially, and central information is gathered over time. Even officially required data can be gathered in this way. However, in order to exercise judgment, the worker needs the support of the agency, as well as a clear understanding of the extent to which the system can be flexible. Whatever the pacing, relevant members of the network should be included early enough so that they understand their important role in the work at hand, and so that the staff can proceed on the basis of an enlarged set of possibilities.

What to Cover

There are three primary goals for intake interviews. *First*, the staff must convey the agency's family-oriented point of view and conduct the meetings so that the family understands its central role. *Second*, they must impart information that the clients will need and obtain the information that's officially required. And, *third*, they must assess the family, looking for problems and conflicts, repetitive patterns, and strengths and resources, as well as preparing the way for continuing family involvement.

These goals overlap, and the staff is usually conveying an attitude, imparting or gathering essential information, and assessing family patterns all at once. Everything we have discussed in earlier sections is relevant to the question of how to do this: a broad concept of family, an interest in the family's perspective, a respectful attitude, an orientation toward strength, and the development of skills for observing, listening, and encouraging family interactions. It's useful, however, to discuss the details, and we do so in the following sections.

Communicating the Need for Family Involvement

The invitation of the family to intake meetings is the first communication about the agency's point of view. It's a powerful message, establishing the priorities in very concrete terms. While one might expect families to be gratified, they're sometimes startled or confused. If they've been through the system before, they're already veterans, trained to travel the same pathways to which most workers are accustomed. They don't expect to be involved in the planning and delivery of services, and need more explanation. The approach of the agency must make sense, particularly since it will involve time and effort. There are many reasons why family members may not respond when invited to participate, and the staff must have a repertoire of mechanisms for communicating the rationale and importance of this policy.

The staff is a step ahead when the identified client is a child. Most families feel responsible for their child, even if they also feel angry or defeated or relieved to be turning the child over to professionals. When James and his mother appeared at the residential center, the first discussion should have conveyed very clearly that the center cannot change the behavior of a young boy by itself, that the family is the most powerful force in the child's life, and that the staff can only help by working closely with family members. Rather than calming the family with reassurances that the child is now in good hands, it's important to preserve the sense of urgency and to convey the need for the family's continuous involvement.

Different situations and ages require other details. When a pregnant teenager comes into a residence, the intake worker may face an angry family. The family may feel that they have lost control over this adolescent, that she got what she deserved, and that they're giving up on her. But she's young and vulnerable, and people in her world may be concerned for her. It's often not difficult to corral a family around the reality that there will be a new baby in the family, and that involvement of the extended family in planning and support is essential.

Intake at a foster care agency is another matter. Everything in the process of removal, court action, and placement has already suggested that the biological family is out of the loop. It's the task of the foster care worker to underline the continuing rights and responsibilities of the child's family, conveying the message that an infant like Wanda must bond with her mother while she remains in care, or that the secure development of an older child depends on continuing contact with his family during the period of placement.

With adult clients, the family may be estranged or critical, or may assume that each adult must handle housing, treatment, or detox programs on his or her own. In justifying the request for family involvement, the worker has two main arguments: first, that family support is an important component of treatment, and second, that changes in the client will have an impact on family life. The intake worker may know, for instance, that a mother's investment in her children will provide the most powerful incentive for abstinence from drugs, and he discusses this immediately with the grandmother, who has custody of the children. He helps her understand that family participation will be an important part of the drug treatment, increasing her daughter's chances of improvement. The worker also discusses the implications of change: The client's improvement will bring about a reorganization of relationships and living arrangements that will affect everybody, and the family needs to work on this together. Hope and logic are communicated at the same time.

In all these situations, the worker is hooking the family into the beginning of the process and laying the groundwork for their continuing participation. To do this effectively requires some of the skills discussed earlier. The worker must convey the conviction that family involvement is crucial for progress and that it's an agency ground rule, but the message is only effective if combined with an emphasis on family strengths. If the worker can convey respect for the family's concern and knowledge, as well as a clear position that the experts cannot do it alone, the family will usually accept the rationale for their participation.

Exchanging Information and Assessing the Family

Even with family members assembled and some understanding established, it's often difficult for workers to change the usual procedures. They may feel obliged to complete the intake forms, a task that may take up the entire first meeting. If that happens, the family assumes the agency has an official understanding of the problem and family members are only present to hear what the program has to offer and comply with bureaucratic requirements. These passive activities reinforce the conception that the agency is taking over.

A family-oriented intake needs to follow a different procedure, one in which the family takes an active role in identifying problems and working toward solutions. It's useful for the worker to approach this interview with some skepticism about the official information in the case folder—checking facts with the family, suspending opinions, and looking for a richer picture of the family's reality. During this kind of intake, the worker focuses on information that only the family can provide, such as the opinions of various members about the nature and origin of their problems and their views about possible solutions. What do they expect from their involvement with the agency? What has been their experience with previous interventions? As a family, do they share an agenda or are they pulling in different directions? At times the worker moves out of the center, allowing for enactments of family style and functioning so she can assess family patterns.

If James, his mother, and his stepfather had participated in this kind of intake, the residential center would have been well on its way to working productively with the boy and his family. The worker might have learned how each parent sees the origin and history of James's violent behavior, how he sees his place in the family vis-à-vis his sister ("the good one"), what the parents resent and accept about the school's complaints, and what happens when James's restless tapping on the arm of the chair disturbs the conversation. The worker would have had the opportunity to comment on the family's concern for the child, noting in particular their wish to manage disagreements, control James, and stay together.

Because intake forms guide so much of staff thinking and effort, it's advisable for an agency to review the forms they traditionally use and to create guidelines that facilitate a family orientation. In the extensive literature on family therapy, there are many examples of the first approach to a family, including the early work of Haley (1976), and, in a later chapter of this book (Chapter 7), we describe a four-step model for family assessment that is often useful. However, there are particular realities that must also be taken into consideration when a family comes to an agency, including not only the problems and strengths of client and family but also prior experience with service systems and expectations for future interactions. In that situation, the intake form must take account of these different aspects.

In Appendix 4.1, we offer an example of questions that might be included in such a form at an agency where children are the primary clients. The items direct attention to family characteristics, concerns, experiences, and expectations—for example, who's in the extended family, how the family is affected by the child's problems, what the family considers the most important focus for help, what solutions they have already tried, what experiences they have had with service systems, how they expect to be involved, and how they describe family stressors and strengths.

Naturally, each agency has its own needs and constraints, and must create or adapt its own forms. However, if the family is seen as a source of information and a resource for further work, intake forms will embody that orientation.[1]

At some point, of course, the worker must gather the historical information that satisfies agency, system, and insurance guidelines on record keeping, and must impart practical information to the clients. Official data often can be gathered late in the session, after a collaborative system of family and agency has been established, or even at subsequent meetings, but the first session cannot finish before the family learns some important facts about the agency. They need to understand how things work, what's special about this program as compared to programs they have known in the past, and what rules and regulations, such as the mandatory reporting of suspected child abuse, determine the freedom of interaction between staff and families. If intake workers can postpone delivering this information until they've learned something about the family and established a relationship, they're in a better position to pinpoint areas where the agency may be relevant to this family's needs. Rather than presenting a litany of available services, the worker can make focused observations and recommendations that go something like "In your situation . . . ", or "Do you think this kind of service would be important for you?", or "I think you should look into this. We can help, if you're interested", and so forth.

Workers from referring or associated agencies may be especially useful for imparting information during intake, or for reviewing past and present services. The counselor from James's school, for instance, might describe conditions for his readmission and services available at that time. However, the intake worker has the responsibility for maintaining the tone of the session, directing the discussion of issues, and keeping the constructive involvement of the family in the foreground.

Laying the Groundwork for Continuous Family Involvement

Intake almost always terminates in a plan for continuing service, no matter what the staff orientation. If the agency is family oriented, intake should move toward a preliminary "contract"—an understanding with the family concerning its future relationship with the agency. In a residential center, the contract might include an agree-

---

[1]See Chapter 7 for the description of a service that used official intake forms as mandated, but inserted family-oriented follow-up questions at relevant points.

ment about the frequency of family sessions, the availability of family members when crises arise that involve the child, and the responsibility of the staff to keep the family informed about treatment
procedures and details of the child's life within the center. In a foster
care agency, the focus might be on the frequency and location of the
biological family's visits with the child, the ways in which the two
families will maintain ongoing contact, and the means for ensuring
that the family will participate in important matters, such as medical
appointments, birthdays, and school functions. In a drug rehabilitation clinic, the family might be asked to provide support for the
recovery efforts of the client, and to participate in multifamily groups
designed to facilitate the reentry of the ostracized member.

NURTURING THE PARTNERSHIP
AND MOVING THE FAMILY ON

If the process of intake has been successfully managed, the client and
family emerge energized and connected to the agency, but the ensuing
weeks and months are a time of potential drift. The danger is that
agency and family will settle into parallel routines that don't require
very much interaction. It's up to the staff to keep things vital; the initiative must come from the agency, which needs to find ways to reach
out to families and keep them involved.

Outreach

Nurturing the relationship with families may require some simple
institutional changes, such as modifying the setting to provide pleas-
ant and inviting public spaces, or expanding center-based activities to
include family members. However, continuing contact also requires
direct outreach, as well as specific efforts to handle developments
that suggest family resistance rather than drift.

Direct outreach should be specific to the case. The worker
knows that James's parents are busy people and have other children.
As time goes by, one or the other misses occasional meetings, and
neither thinks to inquire about James's behavior in the unit or his
educational progress. It's up to the worker to phone them at intervals, conveying the staff's conviction that of course the parents

would be interested and that they have the right to know the details of how James is doing.

Or consider Laura, a new mother living without her child and aware of the judgment that she's not yet a fit parent. She doesn't expect to be included in matters that affect her baby, and it probably wouldn't occur to the foster parents to invite her along when they take Wanda to the doctor for a checkup. Nor would they feel they have the right to do so without agency permission. The worker, however, can make that suggestion to both families, planting a new idea and nurturing the connection between them. An invitation to go along on visits to the doctor slows down the mother's drift away from an infant she hardly knows. It enables her to keep up with her child's development, to have her questions answered, and to prepare for the time when the baby will be released to her care. Expeditions of this kind build shared experience among the network of adults concerned with the infant.

Some forms of outreach can become general policy. In one center for pregnant adolescents, the staff instituted a practice of calling the family twice a week, not to discuss problems or administrative issues but just to touch base. In most situations, parents become used to the idea that they're contacted only when their child is in trouble. A phone call just to talk and exchange information comes as a surprise at first, but then serves to keep open the lines of communication.

If an agency staff thinks together about the practical ways of maintaining contact with families, they will probably come up with a variety of ideas that can be implemented and codified. Consider the following examples, taken from clinics, foster care agencies, residential centers, and day treatment programs. They are actually applicable across the board.

An agency may modify its space. In one foster care agency, a cluster of cubicles was transformed into a room large enough to accommodate several children and the members of both their biological and foster families. In another agency, the boardroom was taken over during certain periods for that purpose. In a day treatment program for drug-dependent mothers, space on the unit was allotted for cribs and toys so the children could be close to their parents while they participated in the program. In a residential center, the furniture in the meeting room was rearranged so that families could mingle informally with the staff. The details vary, but the common theme is the flexibility to experiment with an environment in order to create a family-friendly setting.

Other examples concern program organization. Many facilities offer parenting classes to the identified clients, but several have expanded their boundaries, encouraging companions, spouses, siblings, and grandparents to attend as well. In some settings, it has become customary to hold family meetings before and after a weekend at home in order to process the events that have occurred during that time. Some residential centers have invited family members to come by to discuss incidents that have occurred on the unit, and, in some cases, they have even been welcomed to sit in on a staff review of the case. Of course, new procedures require more than energy and creative ideas on the part of the workers. They also require active participation by the administration, especially if there are to be physical changes in the setting, or a reorganization of staff time and activities.

Outreach to the family may be insufficient as a means of increasing contact. Sometimes the primary clients resist the involvement of their families, either anticipating that family members will cause them grief or because they feel defensive and ashamed. The worker can move slowly but need not give up. It's often possible to bring family issues into the discussion, finding ways to underscore their relevance, detoxify the idea of family involvement, and prepare the groundwork for an actual meeting.

The work with Barbara is such an example. She refused to invite her mother and sister to joint meetings at the drug rehabilitation clinic, arguing that she needed to stand on her own two feet and that her relatives' critical attitude would complicate matters. The counselor was certain from their initial contact, however, that these people were central in Barbara's life and would be important participants in the coming struggle to become free of drugs. She devoted some individual sessions to an exploration of Barbara's family relationships. Whenever Barbara brought up the usual topics that had been occupying previous counseling sessions—her tendency to get involved with violent men, her vulnerability to temptations of drugs, her feelings of being mistreated by the foster care agency that had custody of her children—the counselor would methodically interweave her mother and sister into the discussion. What did they think about Barbara's boyfriends? How did they relate to men? Did they also miss Barbara's children who now were in foster care?

This approach led to the unsurprising revelation that Barbara felt rejected by her mother, was jealous of her sister, and yearned to repair her relationship with both of them but didn't know how. Once this emotional connection became evident, Barbara herself concluded that it might be a good idea to attempt a rapprochement. The family was invited in for a series of sessions, in which some tensions were resolved and Barbara developed a stronger sense of family support. After that, the counselor found a variety of ways to keep the family connected, encouraging Barbara to call her sister when there were things to chat about, suggesting that Barbara invite her family to events at the clinic, and helping to set up an arrangement allowing Barbara's children to visit at their grandmother's house, so that she could see them and the family could be together.

When family members begin to miss scheduled visits with their children, as in the case of James's parents, the staff is faced with a dilemma. If they patiently accommodate to a pattern of no-shows and keep scheduling appointments for "same time next week," they convey a sense that such behavior is expected and doesn't matter all that much. But if they focus on the parents' lack of responsibility, they end up in the position of prosecutors, leaving the family in the complementary position of defendants.

In such situations, the procedures chosen must strike a delicate balance. The worker pursues the family with enough persistence to emphasize the importance of their presence, but without creating antagonism. Most of all, the message must stress one basic fact: The child and staff need their help in order to make satisfactory progress. It's a litany, but it's also the truth, and that fact should lend conviction to the worker's efforts.

In some situations, it's helpful to use the phone or to communicate by letter or e-mail, if that's appropriate, so that contact is maintained. In such cases, the worker mentions the issues being discussed with the child while reinforcing the importance of family participation in the resolution of these problems. She might suggest to James's parents, for instance, that they really need to hear his view of how he's picked on as compared to his sister, and how only they can straighten out his mistaken ideas about their opinions. It also is useful to reschedule missed appointments for the next day, or as soon as possible, rather than waiting for the usual time to roll around.

When foster care workers reach out to the child's biological family, they face a particularly complex dilemma stemming from the requirement to monitor parental behavior. That's part of their job description, and cannot be waived by the leadership of the agency because it originates at higher levels of power—such as protective services and the courts. Workers feel they must demand explanations for acts of noncompliance, such as missing scheduled visits, because, as they have often been told, "The judge will want to know." Under such circumstances, the partnership between agency and family may fall victim to a power struggle, with little energy or disposition to collaborate on behalf of the child.

When the agency is expected to monitor parent behavior, the protection of the partnership may require both an acknowledgment of the staff role as agents of control and some way of distinguishing between that role and the partnership function. In some agencies, it has been possible to organize the staff in teams of two people; one works on compliance with the official mandates while the other is free to focus on enhancing the relationship between agency and family. Because many agencies are constrained in their staffing possibilities, one worker may have to wear both hats. In a particular agency, the worker took to actually wearing hats of different colors, switching them in the middle of the meetings. Though we've said little about the use of humor, metaphor, or playfulness in these chapters, they often carry the day, reducing tension for both staff and family and providing images that help form a bond between them.

Visiting the Family at Home

Outreach usually involves bringing a family into the agency, but it's sometimes useful to maintain contact through a visit. Home visits require sensitivity to the wishes and reactions of the family. It's important for the family to understand that the staff really wants to know the family better, meet other family members, and understand the nature and environment of daily life. Families are often empowered by meeting in their own setting, but are also sensitive to intrusion and to criticism of their lifestyle. It hardly needs mentioning that the worker must enter with respect, and that the purpose of the visit should be contact and communication.

The kind of interchange that takes place depends on the relationship already established. A skilled worker may deal with conflict as it arises, or choose to bypass a discussion in favor of handling the matter at another time. It's almost always preferable to work on family tensions when the primary client is also at home, but there may be times when that's not essential. If a child is caught in the middle of repetitive marital conflicts, for instance, the worker may want to handle that issue during a home visit when the child is absent. Again, that's an informed call by the worker making the visit, and the decision depends both on the situation and the worker's skill.

In residential centers, the question of home visits for the client is an important matter. Visits are essential: They keep the family connected, and provide realistic current material for ongoing work, whether the problems concern tension between the parents and child or the relapse of an adult into substance abuse. Visits also provide a "dry run" for the later reunion of the family. Agency policy, however, is not always benign. Sometimes agencies use visits as part of a reward-and-punishment philosophy rather than seeing visits as part of the problem-solving process.

The curtailment of home visits should be rare, invoked only when a visit to the family home poses a safety risk. Granting or withholding a weekend pass should never be used as a reward or punishment for behavior on the ward, and home visits for a foster child should not be contingent on parental compliance with other aspects of the treatment plan. There's little evidence that these controlling procedures modify negative behavior, but they do convey the message that complying with institutional rules is more important than maintaining family connections.

If incidents occur during home visits and are tense but not dangerous, the worker can place the incident within the context of the evolving relationship among client, agency, and family. Conflicts can be accepted as normal phenomena, to be expected among people who are trying to adjust to each other while living apart. In effect, every visit involves a series of transitions for client and family. The family must expand their patterns of behavior to include the client, and then reorganize again when the visit is over. The client must adapt to family realities after adjusting to expectations in the ward, then readapt to the routines of the institution. That's not easy, and should be discussed as a normal but difficult phenomenon when the family meets with the worker.

Moving On: Discharge and/or Reunification

Finally, there is the matter of "moving on." Discharge from the services of a particular agency creates a period of transition, with all the uncertainty and discomfort accompanying any change, even if the move is positive. Paradoxically, agency supports often dwindle and disappear exactly at this point of increased vulnerability. The case is removed from the worker's roster, which is immediately filled with new clients.

In order to reduce the number of situations where discharge doesn't work, an agency would do well to modify discharge procedures so that attention is intensified. Successful transitions depend on preparatory, carefully processed encounters involving the people and situations that the client will be facing, whether family members, a new foster home, a halfway house, or a different agency. Clients need to experience the next setting, knowing that this is where they will be living, and the people in that setting must prepare for their entry or reentry. Adaptation is a process, evolving through the period before, during, and after the actual transition.

The organization of agency procedures should provide staff time for preparing the transition and for helping clients and families afterward. When Wanda returns to her mother's care, Laura and her boyfriend need the help of a familiar worker to get them through the first adjustments. When Angela finds housing and her husband joins the family at home, workers at the shelter need to help with the move, or put them in contact with people who can be available. And when James returns home, the family needs both preparatory visits and follow-up sessions in order to deal with their apprehension and reinforce the patterns they have been developing for living together.

Such efforts must be a matter of agency policy. The extra sessions in preparation for change require agency approval. The continuing involvement of a worker in the lives of a family after official discharge requires an understanding that this is part of the worker's caseload for a period of time. The implementation of such a policy may be facilitated if the agency understands that this is probably the most economical way to service a family, reducing the likelihood that they will fail to adapt and return through the revolving door. Some percentage of an agency's clientele will move on as a result of improvement and because the staff believes they can make a go of their lives when they leave the agency. It's tragic to undermine that potential by an abrupt and unsupported transition during the last stage of the process.

Appendix 4.1. Suggested Questions for a Family Intake[2]

Identifying Information

Who is in the family?

(If information is not volunteered, ask about family members beyond the child and parents: grandparents, siblings, aunts and uncles. Ask also about people who may be important although they are not kin, such as god-parents. If possible, ask the informants to make a family map.)

The Child's Problems

Why is the child here? What does the family think the reason is, and are there some family members who have different opinions?

When did the problems first appear? What else was happening in the child's life and in the family at that time?

Who else has been affected by the child's problems? How?

What solutions have been tried?

What has been the involvement of child welfare, or of the medical, court, or school systems, in working with the child and family? Has that been helpful?

(If the child has not been described as having problems but has been placed in the care of the agency because of family difficulties, focus the questions on child characteristics, development, and relationships, as viewed by the family.)

The Family: Strengths and Stresses

What are the family's strengths?

(Spend time on this area. If information is not volunteered, ask about support systems, coping mechanisms, qualities the family is proud of, such as family loyalty, resilience, mutual respect, protection and education of the children, and so forth.)

What are the stresses?

(Consider social and economic factors, such as unemployment, racial prejudice, homelessness, limited education, migration, and language difficul-

---

[2]The questions are adapted from a form developed by Ema Genijovich. They are intended as a supplement to questions required by the agency or necessary for official purposes.

ties, as well as personal and family factors, such as illness, drug or alcohol dependence, a death in the family, divorce, and marital tension.)

Family Expectations and Roles

What do members of the family want from the agency? What do they hope will be accomplished? What do they think is the most important concern to focus on first?

Since family members are an important part of the agency's work with the child, which family members should be attending all the meetings?

How might the agency contact family members who don't usually become involved but might be a valuable resource?

PART II

Implementing a Family-Oriented
Model in Service Systems

CHAPTER FIVE

Substance Abuse
A Family-Oriented Approach
to Diverse Populations

It is a basic assumption in the treatment of substance abuse that addiction is a problem of mind and body combined. Because of that assumption, many programs go beyond detoxification and maintenance to include such social and psychological features as group participation, mentoring, or counseling. What has generally not broadened, however, is the focus on the individual and the addiction. Most programs maintain that participants must resolve their problem with addiction before taking on the rest of their lives—much like recovering from the flu or a coma.

Certainly, there have been notable exceptions. Treatment approaches that include family have been described and studied, particularly, though not exclusively, in relation to adolescent drug users (see Liddle & Rowe, 2006; Stanton & Heath, 2004; Szapocznik, Hervis, & Schwartz, 2003; and reviews in Nichols & Schwartz, 2004). The studies have suggested that such programs can be effective, especially if the approach is multisystemic and multidimensional (see Henggeler, Schoenwald, Borduin, Rowland, & Cunningham, 1998, and the Multidimensional Family Therapy (MDFT) model of

Liddle and his colleagues (Liddle, 2002). Nonetheless, most of the treatment for this widespread problem continues to focus on the individual.

The general principles of our family-oriented approach have been described in earlier chapters of the book, and they would apply in a variety of situations where people are under treatment for substance abuse. Each group of drug-dependent clients has its own characteristics, however, and the differences are important for the application of an effective program. The nature of life circumstances, the process that has brought clients into treatment, and the relationship of clients with people affected by their addiction are all relevant. Recovery is a struggle, and the chances of success increase when a program takes account of the specific needs and realities of the client group.

The programs presented in this chapter concern two groups that are very different from each other: on the one hand, the program has been developed for drug-dependent adult women who are pregnant and poor, have multiple problems, and are served by public institutions; on the other, the program is directed at drug-dependent adolescents, both male and female, who come from a variety of socioeconomic circumstances and whose families have placed them in a private residential center for treatment of their addiction. Drug-dependent women living under these conditions and adolescents living in residential centers are almost never offered family-oriented treatment for their addictions, and in this sense, both programs are unusual. The process of consultation and training is different in these two situations, however, because of differences in the clients and in the agencies that serve them.

The program for substance-dependent pregnant women is described first, and has been cowritten with David Greenan. The discussion carries the account from the initial years of consultation and training, first described in the previous edition of this book, through more recent periods and subsequent developments. Description of the family-oriented model for treating adolescents in residential centers is new in this edition, and has been cowritten with Richard Holm. In each case, the aim is to present the family-oriented program, the evolution of the intervention, and the process of facing and resolving problems. The summary in the final section, based on the experience in the two programs, describes the factors that helped this new approach to survive.

THE PERINATAL PROGRAM
with David Greenan

The family-oriented program for women who are poor, pregnant, and chemically dependent has endured for more than 10 years. Introduced into an institution that had no orientation to such an approach, it is remarkable that the essentials have survived. The trajectory has not been smooth, however; the scope and content have shifted with changing circumstances. Since any new approach must face challenges and slippage over time, it's useful to track how the program was adapted in the face of new realities so that the basic intent of helping the women and their families could be maintained.

Phases of the Program and Basic Questions

There have been two phases in the history of this work. The first involved the introduction of a family-oriented program into a hospital-based therapeutic community for drug-dependent adults. The second phase began with a change of venue. Responsibility for the program moved to the Obstetrics and Gynecology (Ob/Gyn) Department within the same hospital as the therapeutic community.

When the perinatal program was first introduced, the therapeutic community was already well established within the Psychiatry Department of a large urban hospital. The community was populated predominantly by male clients, and it had its own rules and procedures. It was almost inevitable that the introduction of a special program for pregnant women, together with a family-oriented training team, would bring the issue of gender to center stage, and would challenge the established procedures.

That situation brought about a series of questions:

How should the staff handle the issues that arise when pregnant women are brought into a predominantly male setting, and how would their decisions be shaped by the training?

What changes would occur in the program when the first babies were born?

Would the perceptions and attitudes of the women be affected by their participation in the program?

Would the family-oriented approach create an impact on other departments and personnel of the hospital?

The second phase began when the program was moved to the Ob/Gyn Department—a move made necessary by the loss of financial support at the original venue. Here there were new questions:

> What made it possible to integrate a family orientation into the services of this department with relative ease?
> What aspects continued, what disappeared, and what developed further?
> How did the consultant and staff adapt the program to changing realities?

These questions, along with some emergent answers, reappear in later sections of the chapter. We begin, however, by considering the first setting for the program and the evolution of the intervention.

The First Setting: The Therapeutic Community as Host

For a reader, as well as a trainer or consultant, an important first step is to understand the context for the introduction of a new approach. The reception will be different, inevitably, if new concepts and procedures are offered to a recently formed staff than if they are brought into an organization where philosophy and services are well established. In this case, the family-oriented program was introduced into an established therapeutic community for substance-abusing clients. Settings of this kind are relatively common in drug treatment centers, and the description can be read as an example of such communities.

The Host Culture

The therapeutic community was located at a day treatment center for chemically dependent adults. Housed within a large urban hospital, the clinic combined a self-help strategy with an array of medical, psychotherapeutic, educational, and social work services. The population was predominantly male, poor, African American or Latino. Candidates, who were often veterans of other drug programs, had to be willing to follow detoxification procedures, maintain abstinence, and remain in attendance to complete the full 18-month program of treatment.

The first stage required attendance 5 days a week and included an intense program of activities, such as 12-step seminars, stress and relaxation workshops, relapse prevention and weekend process meetings before and after the 2-day recess, encounter sessions that challenged members concerning their behavior in the community, and individual contacts with counselors and sponsors. Involvement in the program and sustained sobriety were recognized by an expansion of responsibilities within the community and, in time, a shift to the "reentry" stage, which required attendance only 2 or 3 days a week. During the reentry phase, the focus expanded to a consideration of issues in the outside world—work, family, housing, and so forth. By the time of graduation from the program, the client was expected to be in school, already employed or in job training, and willing to maintain some relationship with the community, such as serving as sponsor for a new client.

The perinatal program was introduced into this community by the director of the hospital's addictions section, who had obtained outside funding to integrate pregnant and postpartum women into the therapeutic community.[1] The combination of medical, psychological, and social services was considered relevant to the multiple problems of the new population, and it was thought that female addicts with outside family ties would find the day treatment structure attractive. A program coordinator and one counselor were added to the staff, and our training center was invited to help with the "family component" of addiction in this new population; namely, the impact of chemical dependency on the family, and the effect of the family on the individual.[2]

Introducing a Family Orientation into the Perinatal Program

The consultants who entered this situation had a long-term goal: to move the staff toward thinking about families and including family members in their work with clients. Any consultant needs to begin, however, by exploring how the system functions and by demonstrating the usefulness of the new approach in concrete ways.

---

[1] We wish to thank Marc Galanter, MD, Director of the Addictions section; Michelle Allen, MD, Director of Ob/Gyn; and Ilene Cohen, PhD, Chief Psychologist of the hospital, for their support during this project.

[2] Salvador Minuchin and Jorge Colapinto were the consultants in the early stages of the project. David Greenan, EdD, subsequently became Program Director, then the consultant and Program Coordinator in both settings.

GATHERING INFORMATION

The initial process of observation and assessment is analogous to the way a family therapist "joins" a family, making an effort to understand their way of doing things before attempting to initiate change. In this situation, the consultants began by talking with staff members and attending meetings at which administrative issues were discussed, policies reviewed, and client behavior evaluated. A primary fact emerged from these meetings: There was almost no reference to families. Clients were discussed in terms of individual success or failure, their relationship to the community, and their interactions with staff.

It became clear that the therapeutic community functioned on the basis of two primary tenets: first, that clients must focus on themselves and deal with their addiction before they do anything else, and second, that the community is the healing context. Everything that occurred in the community was considered part of the struggle for a drug-free life, and relationships among members were seen as the crucial force for personal mastery.

Because addiction was the problem and the therapeutic community the solution, other parts of the client's life were treated as secondary. One client was confronted for arriving late because she stopped at the church on her way to the center, and another, who worked nights as a baker, was urged to give up his job so he could participate fully in the daytime activities of the community. When the consultants asked about the clients' families, they were told they were nonexistent ("Joe doesn't have a family"), rejecting ("Paul's family doesn't want to be bothered"), rejected ("Dave doesn't want his family involved"), or toxic ("Brenda's mother is a bad influence"). Families were not involved in treatment, though they were seen as a possible resource during the reentry phase, when the client was preparing to leave the community.

From the perspective of the therapeutic community, the women would be expected to follow the standard rules and procedures. Commitment to the program would be paramount, and outside concerns and relationships would be suspended until a woman made progress through the phases of recovery. For the family-oriented consultants, however, it seemed necessary to consider the families as a resource, and to protect connections to children, partners, and kin.

Figure 5.1 illustrates the contrast between the perspective of the

	THERAPEUTIC COMMUNITY	FAMILY SYSTEMS
PRIMARY VALUE	Drug abstinence	Connectedness
ROLE OF FAMILY	Secondary	Primary
	Occasional guest	Full participant
	Resource toward end of program	Resource from the beginning
	Complicates treatment	Is complicated by treatment
	Part of the problem	Crucial to the solution
RESPONSE TO NEW CLIENT POPULATION	Must adjust to community culture	Require specific subculture
RELATIONAL STRUCTURE		

FIGURE 5.1. Alternative approaches to the perinatal program: Therapeutic community versus family systems models.

therapeutic community and that of the family-oriented approach. They differ in their views of the role of the family, their expectations for clients entering the program, and their conception of how client, family, and community are related to each other. They also differ in the extent to which they view abstinence as the primary and sufficient goal for treatment. The consultants were bringing an alternative model into the situation, and they would need to expect that this different approach would create conflict.

FIRST STEPS TO CHANGE: MODIFYING STAFF ATTITUDES AND OBSERVATIONS

The team moved slowly at first. Recognizing the power of an established treatment mode, they did not insist on involving family. The early stage of intervention should provide information about new ideas and offer help with particular cases. In this situation, the team offered didactic presentations about family structure, ethnicity, conflicts, and strengths. They also responded to requests for case consultations.

Discussion of case material provides an opportunity to reframe negative judgments and raise interest in the family as a resource for the client. In one case, for instance, the trainer explored the description that Margo's family had rejected her when she became pregnant. Discussion with the staff brought forth additional bits of information: Margo's aunt was potentially supportive, her sister was not so critical, and her mother was angry at her daughter but was interested in the coming grandchild. In the family interview that followed, the staff saw a more loving response to Margo than most of them expected, chiefly because there had been no indication of support in her case record or her own description of family attitudes. After a number of such consultations, the team could suggest mapping a family as a way of gathering information about who is important in a client's life, who likes or is disappointed in her, who is taking care of her children, and so on.

Case demonstrations also increase alertness to details that usually go unnoticed. Staff began to comment that women who said they wanted nothing to do with their families kept bringing up unfinished business—for instance, resentment at a mother who preferred a sibling or guilt at having disappointed somebody they cared about. The team was asked to provide family counseling for certain clients: for Shirley, who feared she would lose custody of her children to her mother, with whom she had an antagonistic relationship; for Julie, whose boyfriend supported her recovery but was verbally abusive; and for Beth, whose complex network of children, foster parents, and workers pulled her in different directions. In family sessions, it was possible to bring tensions and guilt to the surface, and to mobilize the almost universal need to connect and support. Working with Shirley's family, for instance, the counselor drew first on the underlying affection between mother and daughter; then she asked them to talk together about their disagreements and resentment, the way they triggered each others' reactions, and their basic concern for the children and each other—guiding them to explore the strengths of their relationship and their resources for solutions, as well as their problems.

THE BEGINNING OF PROCEDURAL CHANGES: FOCUSING ON INTAKE

Family consultations were helpful in particular cases, but interventions of this kind do not create a change in policy. Progress toward a more pervasive family orientation tends to be blocked by the structure of formal procedures, such as intake, which generally focus on the individual client and the designated problem. To create a broader view, it's necessary to change the nature of the initial contact.

Suggestions that disrupt habitual procedures are not easily accepted. At the least, the timing must be right. In the case of the perinatal program, the high rate of client turnover provided an opportunity. Attendance was erratic, and women were dropping out. The staff attributed defections to poor motivation and an inability to accept the rules, but they feared, as well, that the project would collapse if enrollment continued to decrease. At this point of "felt need," the team suggested that the situation might improve if key members of the applicant's network were involved at intake as partners. The suggestion was followed by specific guidelines on how to conduct a family intake.

The idea of including families was now acceptable, but there is usually a time lapse between the intellectual acceptance of a family ideology and the establishment of relevant procedures. Because the staff found it difficult to assemble family members, and perhaps because they were unsure of how to work with families, they continued to conduct admission interviews with the applicant alone. The idea took hold in a different way, however. The staff began to incorporate family-oriented elements into the first interview. Together with the new client, they mapped the family, asking about family composition, the quality of important relationships, and the attitudes of different family members toward her addiction and potential recovery. Treatment plans that were developed at intake now specified broader goals. For women who had children in foster care, for instance, plans were developed for maintaining and improving contact with the children, even while they remained in placement. Though families were seldom present at such meetings, interviews of this kind reflected the worker's increased awareness of the client's familial context and the relevance of family for her recovery.

This new emphasis brought its own rewards. The grapevine in the neighborhood had communicated clearly that if you were pregnant and chemically dependent, the hospital would take away your infant at birth. The existence of a program concerned with family connections was reassuring, and the number of women who came into the program increased significantly.

Gender and Family: Procedural and Organizational Changes at the Core

Gender and a family orientation were central features of the intervention, and they represented an intrusion into the established therapeutic community. It was inevitable that the needs and behavior of the pregnant women would challenge the customary way of doing things, and that the interventions of the consultants would create a clash of perspectives. The result was a series of small and larger crises, followed by procedural and organizational changes that were developed to resolve the issues.

RISING TENSION: THE IMPETUS FOR CHANGE

As the program grew, tensions arose within the staff. The women were coming late and taking a less active part in meetings. Core staff of the therapeutic community maintained that it was important to follow the usual disciplinary procedures; the perinatal staff wanted more flexibility in enforcing the rules and responding to violations. In this atmosphere, two perinatal coordinators resigned in rapid succession and David Greenan, trained as a family therapist and associated with our center, became the program director. He served as consultant and coordinator for more than a decade, carrying the program through changes in venue, personnel, and financial support.

With the advent of Greenan, the director position was stabilized, but his activities did not calm troubled waters. He mounted a vigorous recruitment campaign, involving outreach to women's shelters in the area and to the hospital's Ob/Gyn Department. Though the roster of clients grew apace, staff disagreements also increased, and the conflict was brought to the monthly meeting of administrators and staff.

CHANGES IN ORGANIZATION: CREATION OF A DE FACTO SUBSECTION FOR THE WOMEN

During this meeting, the family-oriented team took a clear stand, maintaining that most of the difficulties stemmed from realities associated with gender, and that the perinatal clients should be regarded as a special population. The women had arrived in the community through a different route than traditional clients, having faced the choice of joining the program or losing their infants. They did not live at the hospital-based shelter, as many of the male clients did, and they were usually connected to an outside network of children, friends, and kin. The women were confused by the rules of the larger therapeutic community, which did not favor dealing with family concerns even though caseworkers from elsewhere in the system encouraged the continuation of contact.

After some discussion, a solution was agreed on: The community staff would tolerate differences in the way this population related to the program, and the perinatal staff would develop activities to meet the specific needs of their group. In effect, the perinatal program became a differentiated subsection of the community. The women continued to participate in community activities and were monitored for sobriety and progress, but they were granted more leeway in following rules and allowed to attend activities specifically designed with a family focus.

THE IMPACT OF THE BABIES: AN EXPANSION OF STRUCTURE AND SERVICES

As women in the program began to give birth, a new problem arose: Where would the babies be during the day while the women participated in the program, and who would take care of them? In this situation, workers who were part of the child welfare system disagreed among themselves. Most assumed that the city welfare agency would supply homemakers to care for the babies at home, while others were concerned about the long hours of separation between mothers and their infants. Situations that require a definite decision are like conflicts that have come to a head; they provide an opportunity for recommendations that are clear and logical. In this case, proponents of the family-oriented approach took the position that mother and child, as a unit, should be considered participants in the program. They noted that expert opinion considers the mother–child bond crucial for healthy development, and they suggested that the presence of the babies might enhance recovery rather than acting as an impediment.

The controversy was useful, sparking an examination of policy and involving the chief epidemiologist of the hospital in the decision. He ruled that both healthy babies and those born with positive toxicity could be cared for at the hospital, as long as certain provisos were followed concerning sanitary precautions, there was provision of an adequately furnished area, and so forth. As a result, a large room was set aside for the perinatal group, with cribs, equipment for handling formula, pictures, and toys. The nursery became a "home room," where the mothers could congregate to talk and relax.

NEW STRUCTURES AND INNOVATIVE PROCEDURES: THE ESTABLISHMENT OF FAMILY-FOCUSED DISCUSSION GROUPS

It was the responsibility of the perinatal staff, aided by the consultants, to develop activities of particular relevance for the pregnant women. Mindful of the importance of family concerns for this population, the staff created two new groups: the *parent support group* and the *family issues group*.

The Parent Support Group. All of the women in the program were about to bear a child, and almost all had older children as well. For many, parenting was the core of life. A parent support group was created, and specialists from the Child Life Department of the hospital were invited to organize the activities. Aside from the obvious value of such leadership, the arrangement offered a new model of communication and combined service across traditional, carefully maintained boundaries within the hospital.

Meetings of the parent support group were held in the Child Life nursery of the hospital. The arrangement offered a variety of benefits; some emotional, some informational. The women discussed their concerns as parents with the Child Life staff, and they learned something about the particulars of child development and different ways of stimulating growth. They were also introduced to other services offered by the department, such as the developmental evaluation of infants and toddlers and the therapeutic nursery program.

In time, the parent support group opened up to include fathers and other adults who shared parenting roles with the women, as well as men from the therapeutic community who had asked to participate as fathers. The interest in discussing life issues beyond addiction had spread, in some measure, to the larger community. The effect was to last only as long as the perinatal project remained within that setting, but both the participation of the Child Life specialists and the presence of people from outside the perinatal group were important developments, suggesting that boundaries around a special population should be firm enough to protect their status but sufficiently permeable to allow for useful interaction with others.

The Family Issues Group. This group departed clearly from the traditional concerns of the therapeutic community. The focus was openly on "family," and on problems with outside relationships. Initially filled with expressions of anger, resentment, and conflict, the meetings moved on to explore alternatives and consider solutions. Child custody was a common problem, for instance, and many of the women were most familiar with solutions that involved the courts, estrangement from relatives, and, often, defeat. A watershed occurred when Katherine, a member of the group, was persuaded to invite her aunt in for a discussion. The children had been living with the aunt for several years, and there was tension now about eventual custody. Katherine and her aunt were wary, at the beginning of the meeting, but with the aid of the coordinator they came to understand each other's perspective—the mother's wish to have her children and the aunt's strong attachment formed over the years.

As this adversarial relationship moved towards planning and collaboration, the staff, as well as the clients, began to shift in their understanding of the issues and possible solutions. The goal of reconnecting with family members became central and the effort to repair relationships was seen as a constructive force for recovery.

The Development of Clients as Stakeholders

With time, the women accumulated experience as participants in the groups, and, with initial guidance, some began to lead the discussions. Familiar with neighborhood realities and recurrent personal problems, they became skillful facilitators. In the process, a sense of solidarity among the women grew stronger, and they initiated practical activities to ease the burdens of daily life. They organized an informal co-op, for instance, to care for the children of women who needed time to keep medical appointments, go for job interviews, or attend to family matters. The mobilization of support extended beyond the immediate group, so that when a prospective program participant mentioned that she was facing a hostile environment in her shelter, one of the veterans commented, "They treat you like that because they think you're all by yourself. It's important that they know you're not a lonely person, that you do have a family. And if you don't, we'll be your family." The group then agreed to show up at the shelter, "not to intimidate anybody, but so that they know you're not alone, that we care for you." As they took on more active and varied functions, the women became "stakeholders," in a sense, participating in a program that had become important to them.

Discussion in the two groups expanded, over time, reflecting the fact that mothers and infants were both part of the program. The parent support group now consisted of real dyads, and the Child Life staff worked directly on the sending and receiving of cues between mother and child, on feeding and care, and on understanding the developmental patterns of one's own child. The family issues group focused on the practical implications of motherhood and its connection with other aspects of family life. Questions of support from fathers, partners, extended family, neighborhood networks, and social services became important. The women gathered information and became increasingly skillful at mobilizing available resources.

The Wheel Turns: Approaching Program Termination within the Therapeutic Community

The special grant for the perinatal program lasted for 5 years. As the final period approached, the project was in full swing. The enrollment of new clients was adequate. Veterans were giving birth to healthy babies, continuing to participate as leaders of the flourishing support groups, and serving as role models for uncertain newcomers. The coordinator concentrated on increasing the integration of necessary services. He sought contact with the outside community, including local shelters, solidified the relationship with the Ob/Gyn Department, and instituted multidisciplinary meetings that brought together personnel from a variety of hospital departments.

Some Answers to the Basic Questions

At the end of these 5 years, it was possible to answer some of the questions raised at the beginning of the project. The women had been integrated into the therapeutic community by creating an informal subsection, with activities dedicated to their particular needs. The advent of the babies had led to the acceptance of mother and infant as a combined unit in the program, to the creation of an infant-oriented space, and to a liaison with specialists who worked directly with mother and child. Many of the women had become more self-confident as they participated in the program. They connected with each other, created support groups that reached beyond hospital boundaries, and became stakeholders in the program.

The consulting team had carried a consistent family perspective through this period, and had been able to influence procedures when crises arose and decisions were required. They encouraged modifications in the intake process, the creation of subgroup boundaries that were both firm and reasonably permeable, and the involvement of administrators at higher levels of the system when bold decisions required their approval. The staff had been actively engaged throughout. They struggled with challenges to their customary way of working, provided input from their perspective, and, through family-oriented demonstrations and guidelines, were able to adapt to change.

A question not raised earlier concerns the effect of the perinatal program on the substance dependence of the participants. At the least, it would be important to know that the women did as well in controlling their addiction as other members of the community did. In fact, researchers working in the hospital's Division of Alcoholism and Drug Abuse were able to establish the positive effects of the program on the cocaine addiction of the participants (Egelko, Galanter, Dermatis, & Maio, 1998). In a comparative study, they found that urine toxicology and continuing attendance at the treatment program were significantly improved for perinatal participants in the family-oriented program, in contrast with nonperinatal clients and with perinatal clients who were not in a program concerned with families.

Though there were so many positive indicators, the family-oriented approach was not continued within the therapeutic community when the project concluded. That outcome is not unusual when funds are no longer available, but it was certainly disappointing, particularly since the program was so effective. The aim of an intervention is always to create a change that will last. However, the fact that the family orientation had never spread to the predominantly male population of the community was probably significant. In addition, one might speculate that it was considered too costly to fund the perinatal staff and the baby nursery from within the department budget, that the changes were creating ripples in the community the staff found difficult to handle, and/or that the perinatal population with its multiple needs called for a commitment the department could not take on. Whatever the reasons, such features as the baby nursery and the family discussion groups were phased out. The approach did not disappear from the institution, however. As a result of supporting factors described below, the program moved, in modified form, to the Ob/Gyn Department, where it was integrated into the ongoing services of the department.

Change of Setting: Obstetrics and Gynecology as Host

When the program changed venue, the new department could not maintain all the features developed during the earlier years. Nonetheless, the basic orientation and some family-centered activities were accepted into the new department with relative ease.

The ease of transition was a function of several factors: the relationship already established with the Ob/Gyn Department; the department's positive attitude toward family work; the effort expended by program and department leaders; and the involvement of personnel from other sections of the hospital. In the following section, we summarize these factors. We describe, also, the obstacles that arose along the way, since they typify the forces that threaten the survival of any intervention.

Integration into the New Department: The Provision of Space, Time, and Services

A liaison with the Ob/Gyn Department had been established during the earlier period, and through all the events of subsequent years, the department has remained steadfast in support of a family orientation. The director and predominantly female staff saw the treatment of addiction and recovery as part of a health-driven philosophy. Working in a hospital located among the urban poor, they were familiar with the life conditions of their clientele, and they considered it necessary to adopt a systemic approach. Early on, the staff had set aside one day each week to provide special services in their high-risk clinic for substance-dependent clients. They now took on additional responsibilities. To the extent possible, the department provided space and time for group activities, family sessions, and multidisciplinary meetings. The staff also assumed responsibility for monitoring drug usage through tests of urine toxicology, incorporating this routine into their general reviews of client health. In effect, the department was integrating the approach of the program into the structure of hospital services.

The Support of Family Activities: Groups, Family Sessions, and the Further Exploration of Gender

GROUPS

Family-oriented group meetings continued in the new setting, where they were led by women who were successful veterans of the perinatal program. Coming from life conditions similar to the newcomers, they represented hope for the future. They were drug free, had delivered healthy babies, and were usually living with their reunited families. The group was formalized as a "breakfast club," in which the women discussed parenting skills, supported efforts to remain clean, and organized an expansion into the community as a bulwark against isolation. The veterans of the program, as well as newcomers, continued to function as stakeholders, promoting and implementing the basic ideas of the intervention.

FAMILY SESSIONS

Family sessions were also conducted in this setting when the staff requested help with a particular client. The following case offers a useful illustration, not only because the session was valuable for the woman and her family but also because it affected the issue of gender, expanding the perception and tolerance of the staff toward male members of a woman's family.

Mona came to the Ob/Gyn clinic when she was pregnant with her third child. Her 4-year-old daughter had been placed in foster care soon after birth because of positive toxicity, and her son, Mateos, 2½, was living at home with Mona and Oscar, the father of the unborn child. The couple met when both were clients in the therapeutic community, and both had recovered successfully from their addictions. Now, as Mona was about to give birth to their child, foster care workers had decided that her situation was stable and that her daughter could come home to live with her.

The Ob/Gyn staff referred Mona for therapy because they found her confrontational and hard to handle. What the consultant saw when he met with the family, however, was a severely stressed woman about to give birth, caring for an active toddler, and preoccupied with the return of a child she had never lived with, though she had visited her over the years and loved her dearly.

In the first family session, a repetitive pattern emerged: Mona and Oscar were intensely connected, but the relationship was characterized by Mona's angry attacks on her partner whom she considered lazy and untrustworthy, Oscar's accusation that she was focused completely on the children, and efforts by Mateos to divert them. The therapist interrupted the shouting, pointing to the effect on Mateos and highlighting the fact that Mona was trying to function as "Superwoman." Probing the possibility of enlisting Oscar's aid, he asked Mona, "Can you let Oscar help you . . . ? Do you let him take care of Mateos?" He then suggested that Oscar take care of the boy while he talked with Mona. The child went contentedly to Oscar, who turned out to be, as Mona admitted, a "natural." He related to children easily, drawing on the skills developed in the large Hispanic family of his childhood.

As therapy continued, the therapist focused on challenging Oscar's peripheral role in the family, alleviating Mona's tendency to take everything on herself, and releasing Mateos from his ineffectual role as peacemaker. The couple talked about their changing perceptions of each other, and about altering the pattern of responsibilities in the family. In the final session before their child was born, they said they had decided not to take the little girl back from foster care. Though it was a sad and difficult decision, they knew she was settled and happy, that the foster family loved her, and that, with this decision, they would be better able to ensure a stable environment for Mateos and the new baby.

GENDER: A CHANGE IN ATTITUDES TOWARD MALES

It was a simple case for a family therapist, concerning two people who cared for each other and involving neither violence nor current drug use. For the staff, however, it was a turning point. The perception of Mona changed, and, equally important, they saw her partner as a resource for her well-being and that of the children. Staff attitudes and policies, to that point, had been protective. Strongly committed to their patients and aware of past abuse in many cases, the staff had not allowed male members of a woman's family on the premises. Following this case, however, with its reframing of the issues and its satisfactory resolution, attitudes softened. Now, women were allowed to invite family members, including male partners, into the ward, and fathers were encouraged to be present at the time of birth. This profound change of policy was similar, in a sense, to the acceptance of mother and child as the participating unit in the therapeutic program when the babies were born. In each case, an understanding of the relevant system expanded: from mother to mother plus child in the earlier situation, and from mother and child to the threesome of mother, father, and child in this new setting. That broader understanding brought with it the possibility of added attention and service for all the participants.

As part of this new attitude, the women's support group accepted family members, and women who had delivered healthy babies came to the group accompanied by fathers as well as children. Discussions concerning relationships reflected the views of both partners, and questions about child rearing included the experience of functioning together as parents. The exploration of gender issues that had begun within the therapeutic community became more differentiated, allowing the staff and their clients to make case-based judgments about the advantages and risks of including male members of the family in prenatal care and the birth process.

Multidisciplinary Involvement: Outreach and Case Conferences

Multidisciplinary case conferences had been initiated by the consultant in order to coordinate services for each woman and to extend the understanding of family as a resource. The first meetings brought together personnel involved with particular cases, but, in time, the conferences broadened to include key personnel around the hospital. Here, the social and political skills of the Ob/Gyn medical director were crucial. She made the contacts that were necessary for producing collaboration rather than resistance to this way of working. The hospital's chief social worker and chief psychologist were invited, along with pediatricians, child welfare workers, obstetricians, nurses, and drug treatment staff.

As part of the same effort to involve a broader band of hospital staff, the consultant made himself available for a variety of services. He conducted grand rounds for Ob/Gyn residents, presented talks concerning families and children, and was available for case consultations and family sessions. Following this combination of outreach and multidisciplinary conferences, attitudes began to change. References to "crack moms" and "snow babies" diminished, and the circle of supportive personnel from other departments widened.

The Role of Leaders

The perinatal program was originally introduced into the therapeutic community by the director of the addictions section, whose efforts secured the grant for this unique work. Continuation in the new department became possible through the support of the Ob/Gyn Department's medical director. She facilitated the provision of space and time, worked with her staff as they took on new functions, and brought her administrative skills to bear on the effort to involve personnel from other areas of the hospital.

As the coordinator of the family program, the consultant faced two major issues when the program moved from the therapeutic community to the new department: whether to curtail or expand his activities, and what stance to take when his work could not be funded. He opted for a very active role, involving case conferences, teaching, consultation, and outreach into the hospital and community. During periods without funding, he continued to offer service. That decision is a matter of personal choice and practical realities, but the question of whether such bridges are essential to ensure program survival must necessarily be considered. It seems clear that people in executive positions must commit themselves in practical ways if positive changes are to endure.

Obstacles: Finances, Changing Official Policies, and the Unexpected

Almost any administrator or staff member employed in public service can provide examples of obstacles that have obstructed the smooth continuation of their work. In many cases, the examples would involve inadequate funding or changes in official policy, and this situation was no exception.

After the original perinatal grant terminated, funding for family consultations followed an erratic course. The consultant contributed his services until the department received a 3-year grant and applied part of the funds to consultation. The work of the high-risk clinic and the family-oriented program during this period was certainly cost effective, with the high rate of full term, drug-free babies offering a clear contrast to the expense of treating toxic infants. However, when support was no longer available, consultation continued again on a voluntary basis until the chief psychologist of the hospital, in possession of a discretionary grant, assigned funds for 5 years of consultation to the family-oriented program. Her decision was the result of contacts established through the multidisciplinary case conferences and the impact of that experience on hospital staff.

Policy changes at official levels support some programs and threaten others. With respect to pregnant, substance-dependent women, a new mandate issued by the city administration affected core features of the family-oriented approach. The ruling stated that women with drug histories who are at risk for delivering toxic infants must live in residential treatment centers. Since families could no longer be seen at the Ob/Gyn clinic, it became necessary to work directly with the residential facilities, beginning again with basic ideas about families as a resource. Not all residential centers have been receptive, but when the approach has created interest, the center has provided in-service training for staff, as well as encouragement and support for family-focused work.

Sustaining the Effects of an Intervention:
A Preliminary List of Factors

Detailed consideration of the forces that sustain an approach is best postponed until the second program has been described, but we can finish this section by noting the factors that have emerged so far:

- Integration into organizational policies and procedures.
- Leadership commitment.
- The creation and involvement of stakeholders.
- Adaptability.

In presenting the second program, we will be concerned with the question of whether these factors reappear, as well as with noting whether additional factors emerge when the setting and the conditions are different.

THE RESIDENTIAL CENTER FOR ADOLESCENTS
with Richard Holm

Adolescents tend to explore life, though not always in socially acceptable ways, and it's a rare adult who doesn't remember that drugs and alcohol were "around" when they were growing up. For some adolescents, however, the habit takes over. They're in trouble, and when that's recognized, families, school authorities, or the courts take action, sending the adolescent to a therapist, a day program for substance-dependent youth, or a residential treatment center.

Family therapy is not common in the treatment of substance abuse, but there is a growing effort to work with the family when adolescents are involved. Over the last decade or so, carefully designed programs have been developed and applied, and they have demonstrated encouraging results, particularly when the approach is systemic and combines family work with other forms of monitoring and intervention. (See the Multidimensional Family Therapy [MDFT] approach of Liddle and his colleagues [Liddle, 2002]; the Brief Strategic Family Therapy [BSFT] model [Szapocznik et al., 2003]; and the multisystemic model of Henggeler et al., 1998, among others.) These models have generally been implemented in outpatient settings or day treatment centers with families whose adolescent is living at home. There has been little attempt to introduce a family orientation into residential centers for substance-dependent adolescents.

In this section of the chapter, we describe the experience of introducing a family-oriented program into a residential center. The basic principles are similar to those that have been implemented effectively in outpatient therapy, but the context is different. In a residential setting, it's necessary to consider organizational structures and staff attitudes, as well as the teaching of skills for family work. Our aim here is to describe the process of training and to consider the kinds of questions that were raised in the prior section:

> What changes occurred in the organization or procedures at the residence?
> How were families included?
> How did the consultant and staff handle issues that arose during the training?
> What factors blocked or sustained the new approach?

The Host Culture

The family-oriented program was introduced into a residential center for male and female drug-abusing adolescents between the ages of 13 and 18. The center was part of an established substance abuse treatment organization that administered both community-based and residential facilities for adults and young people.[3] The adolescents came from both lower- and middle-class families and were predominantly, though not exclusively, Caucasian. They were referred by the courts, probation officers, or the school system, and were sometimes brought directly by their parents.

The staff for these 70 adolescents included administrators, directors of the different services, and six counselors. The latter were generally Certified Alcohol and Drug Counselors (CADCs), and some were graduates of the organization's drug rehabilitation program. The clinical director was responsible for assessment and treatment. The residential director supervised the counselors, who ran the encounter groups and were directly responsible for behavioral interventions.

Applicants were screened on the basis of an individual interview, with a parent or guardian present to provide information on drug history and behavior. Families received an information packet, which made it clear that the staff would now serve as the parents and big brothers and sisters for the adolescents in their charge, and that the mission was to deliver a comprehensive treatment program that was multidisciplinary, peer oriented, and cost-effective. The staff, familiar with the approach through personal experience and training, regarded themselves as the "healing family," and functioned in accordance. Families were excluded from this effort, and the activities of the sparsely populated Family Association were considered peripheral.

The residence was basically a therapeutic community, and the activities for participants were similar to those described in the earlier section of the chapter. They included group meetings, encounter sessions, counseling, the monitoring of behavioral compliance with clearly stated rules, established disciplinary procedures, attention to health and abstinence, and, for this adolescent population, schooling.

Within this structure, new residents followed a sequence of levels. When Cara was accepted into the residence, she spent approximately 1 month on the entry level, where she was oriented to the

[3]We wish to thank James Curtin, Administrator, Daytop New Jersey, for his involvement and support throughout the project, and Jennifer Kenny, EdS, Coordinator of Family Therapy, for illustrative material.

program, lived under constant supervision, and was assessed for compliance and behavior. Having adapted well, she moved to the next level, where she was expected to take on more responsibilities within the facility and earned such privileges as off-campus trips and home visits. Success at this level brought her to the reentry phase, where she could follow a more flexible schedule, spend weekends at home, and participate in exploratory activities pointed toward discharge, such as groups focused on relapse prevention. The staff identified an outpatient resource, in preparation for discharge, and indicated the existence of an aftercare program for graduates like Cara who were living in the vicinity. Cara's progress was relatively smooth, but residents like Andreas, who was alternately sulky and rebellious, spent more time at each level, lost and regained privileges, and sometimes dropped out.

This center, then, was implementing a self-sufficient, therapeutic community, following the model of the larger organization to which it belonged. Since that was the situation, we need to consider how the request for family-oriented training came about, and raise an additional question: Would the family-oriented training create changes that could coexist with this established model, or would it alter the customary procedures of the therapeutic community? Looking ahead, we can say that it has done both!

Introducing a Family Orientation into the Residential Program

The search for a family-oriented approach was initiated by the administrator of the area, who had trained as a family worker and was concerned with persistent issues at the facility: that the length of stay was too long, that participants were leaving the program before completion, and that changes were not maintained after discharge. It was a familiar set of problems for residential centers, and the administrator thought that more family involvement would increase the effectiveness of their work.

The administrator selected one residence for a pilot effort and initiated a series of steps to prepare a family-oriented clinical staff. Three members were sent to the Minuchin Center for external training in family work, forming a core group to bring back new information and skills. A coordinator of family therapy was appointed from within the staff, and a series of family case conferences was established for clinical workers. These experiences were profitable but, as they began to work with families, the staff found it difficult to handle conflict or affect family relationships. It seemed evident that they would need on-site supervision, and the administrator approached the Minuchin Center to request an intensive program of consultation and training. The resulting arrangement provided for weekly half-day training sessions, with mandatory attendance for designated staff, to be conducted on site by Richard Holm.[4]

The Process of Training

It's important to note that the program developed for this organization required a different role from the consultant/trainer than that required by the perinatal program. The director of the perinatal program had invited the consultants to work with families of the women, as needed, and to suggest in general how families and addiction might be connected; he did not ask the consultants to train the staff of the therapeutic community, and the changes they were able to introduce into the structure of the treatment were the result of timing and skill rather than an invited role. The arrangement at the residential center, on the other hand, was specifically for staff training. It did not include any intervention into the structure of community activities for the adolescents, but the task of working with staff and administrators was comprehensive. The consultant was invited to teach and supervise, and to be available for discussions about staff procedures and organizational changes that would facilitate constructive contact with the families.

All the chapters in the second half of this book contain descriptions of the training process, and it will probably be useful for readers to note the similarities and differences from one situation to another. Because the training was conducted by professionals who shared an orientation and had often worked together, many elements are similar; but because each organization had particular needs and the consultants had particular styles, there are also differences. We have tried to avoid unnecessary repetition in the descriptions, but have included enough detail so the basic elements of the training in each situation can come through.

---

[4]Richard Holm, DSW, served as consultant and trainer for the first 3 years of the program.

Beginning the Process

In the first meeting with 30 members of the staff, the consultant focused on "joining" and on experiential exercises. After mutual introductions, a free-form discussion about staff concerns included reservations about the training, continuing problems of client drop-out, relapse, and length of stay at the residence, and the need for staff to improve their skills for working with families.

The rest of the meeting consisted of experiential activities, created to promote an understanding of family patterns and a beginning grasp of systemic ideas. One exercise, for instance, focused on family shapes, life cycles, and transitions. Participants created a nonverbal choreography of a family moving from a two-parent household to a one-parent household, then to an intergenerational family, and, finally, to a stepfamily. The experience prompted a discussion of closeness and distance, authority and control, and the difficulties of dealing with the needs of different family members in these varied circumstances. The trainer could then introduce concepts of hierarchy, boundaries, coalitions, and so forth. The meeting finished with videotapes that illustrated and reinforced the concepts.

In the weekly meetings that followed, the consultant faced the effect of mandated attendance: an unspoken division of the staff into those who were motivated and those who were not. In some training situations, it's possible to select motivated staff for a pilot project; in others, such as this one, an administrative order forces the attendance of people who are passive or resistant. It's usually not advisable to challenge the mandate, but it's possible to focus the procedures on participants who are interested, as this trainer did, while the others look on. In a development that was not totally unexpected, the energy and excitement of the central participants reached some of the staff who had not been part of the "coalition of the willing," and they became increasingly involved.

The Structure of the Meetings

It's useful to create procedures that are repeated at each meeting. That gives the participants a sense of predictability that is reassuring. The trainer divided each meeting into three phases. In the first phase, a staff member talked about a family he or she was working with, describing the referral information, mapping the family's structure, subsystems and boundaries, and summarizing relationships both within the family and to larger systems. The presenter then described what he or she was trying to achieve and the difficulties associated with the work. Others who knew the family added their comments, and the group then watched a videotaped session with this family conducted by the presenter. As the session proceeded, the group was to keep in mind what the worker was trying to do and where he or she was stuck. The ensuing discussion focused on family patterns and relationships, guided to include not only problems but also indications of strength, and on the interchange between the worker and family members. The trainer told the staff he wanted them to "catch people doing things right," both in the family and in the work of their colleagues.

The second phase involved role playing. After the participants had assessed the session, volunteers played out a new and different interview. They practiced skills for engaging family members, asking relationship questions, exploring the problem, tracking sequences of behavior, creating enactments to highlight patterns of interaction, and reframing the situation so that parents could assume leadership in the process of problem solving.

In the final phase, the consultant shifted to another level. Building on concrete examples that had already been discussed, he guided the staff toward noticing the parallels between an effective handling of issues with a family and a productive approach to organizational problems at the agency. Sometimes the point was made by extending the implications from family work to the organization, and sometimes the process was reversed. At one meeting, for instance, a counselor remarked that she was having difficulty carrying a dual role—"as surrogate parent with the kids . . . and also as the family worker." She wondered how she could be an authority figure all week, then work in a different way with the family. The consultant turned the question back to the staff: How could they handle this problem?

The discussion clarified the realities that could not be changed in this situation and produced an array of possible options, enabling the counselor to organize clearer boundaries for her work. The consultant pointed out how creative the staff had been in coming up with ideas. As experts on their organization, they had drawn on their own resources and come up with possible solutions. He then commented on the parallels with family work and asked if they could turn problems back to the families in the way he had just done with them. Somebody called him "sneaky" and everybody laughed, but the point was taken. The staff understood that a family will profit from the space and authority to discuss and resolve issues internally, just as an organization can use its own resources to review a situation and create positive changes. The further implication was, of course, that this mechanism would be available to families and organizations after the expert had moved on.

Content: Working with the Family

In the early meetings, the consultant focused on how to engage the families and assess family patterns. In time, he moved to the handling of conflict, and to questions about helping families explore more constructive pathways for coping with problems. Throughout, there was an emphasis on ceding a more central and powerful role to the parents—perhaps the most difficult task of all. With a concept of themselves as the "healing family," the staff were used to functioning *in loco parentis*, as experts and problem solvers. It took some effort for them to realize that this was counterproductive; that it reinforced a conviction on the part of the parents that they were helpless failures, dependent on the competence of those who knew more. The task for the trainer was to help the staff step back, conveying the message at the same time that the parents were crucial partners in the process of fixing their kids, and that they had the resources to do so.

It was a message that needed to come early, as new participants and families came into the program, and the reception was not always smooth. A grateful acceptance by the family is never guaranteed. In one of the cases described more fully below, the idea that parents would be involved came as a welcome surprise. Nan's mother told the worker that in previous programs, "I never knew what was going on with my daughter," and the idea that she would be needed was gratifying. Other families, however, are resistant, either because they have been relieved to turn over the burden of sparring unsuccessfully with their recalcitrant adolescents or because they assume they will be the target of reproach. Bud's father was wary when the worker told him that parents are a key resource in the work at this residence. A veteran of past programs involving Bud's older brother, this father maintained that parents "get blamed by everyone." That's neither a rare experience nor an unreasonable fear. In this case, the worker emphasized that they would be working with the family in search of creative ways to handle the difficulties they were struggling with, and for Bud's father, that formulation made sense.

Two Illustrative Cases

The following cases illustrate the new procedures introduced into the facility, particularly with regard to the inclusion of parents. It should be noted, in connection with these cases, that bringing in family members to participate in disciplinary decisions was unprecedented in this, or any, therapeutic community, affecting the usual structure quite profoundly without interfering with the daily activities.

The Case of Nan

When Mary, Nan's mother, called the residential center, she said that she was "at the end of her rope." Now 15, Nan had already explored a wide variety of drugs, with heroin and marijuana as her drugs of choice. She was failing in school, had completed an outpatient program without effect, and had been ordered into therapy by the court. During the admission procedures, the family counselor interviewed Mary and Nan about the family situation. Mary had been a single parent since Nan's father left the family 12 years earlier, and she had no contact with other family members. Her only source of support was Janet, her partner and close friend, who had lived in the household for a number of years, but moved out when Nan was about 9 because of tension between the child and herself.

This first meeting with the family counselor became chaotic—a seesaw in the struggle for power between a mother and daughter who were close but abrasive. The counselor discussed with Mary how much both the residence and Nan needed her participation if therapy was to be effective, and all agreed to a schedule of regular meetings. Service planning included the behavioral counselors, in keeping with the facility's new emphasis on coordinated interventions, and it was understood that the staff would be working as a team throughout the period of Nan's stay.

The family meetings were crucial, but events that arose at the residence were equally important, allowing the staff to draw Mary into a more effective parenting role. Some events were routine, calling for decisions about Nan's progress and next steps. When Nan had been at the residence for 6 weeks, for instance, the staff called Mary to ask, "Do you think it's time to move her to level 2? Is she ready?" Mary gave her opinion, commented on her reasons, and was part of the decision.

When basic rules were broken, the situation became more complex. Nan had violated one of those rules by having sex with another resident. When Nan was caught, she erupted, demanding to leave the program. The usual procedure was to enforce discipline, while attempting to convince the adolescent to remain in the program. In keeping with the new policies, however, the family counselor called Mary, who asked immediately, "Are you going to discharge her?" The counselor replied with a question: "What do you think we should do? Can you come in and assist us with this?"

At the family meeting, Mary was enraged, telling Nan that she could either change or go to the detention center, ". . . because you're not coming home!" It's important to realize how much support and skillful work had gone on in order to bring Mary to this point of assertion. Stepping back and ceding authority to the parents is not sufficient. The parents have been through this; they have experienced the reality that adolescents are strong and effective adversaries, and by the time their children are in residential treatment, the parents expect to be defeated before they start. As in all work with families in conflict, the counselors need to punctuate the discussions—underlining the points of small success, intervening and redirecting when the quarrel becomes destructive, and supporting the authority of the parents while encouraging them to listen when the adolescent expresses resentment. After a series of meetings, Mary felt confident enough to assert her authority and risk the rejection she feared, while Nan was able to express her anger, admit her mistake, and make the choice to stay at the facility.

In the subsequent period, Mary and Nan worked on discussing expectations about the future. What would be the consequences if Nan violated agreements about behavior during her weekends at home? And what relationships would support Mary when she granted Nan more separation and autonomy? As Nan moved to the reentry level, family meetings began to include Janet, Mary's partner. She would be the primary source of support for Mary in building a full life that did not depend on Nan. Together, they all worked on issues dealing with the authority of the parent, on boundaries among the three, and on conflicts between Nan and Janet, in which Mary served as peacemaker and facilitator of their exchanges.

As Nan prepared to return home, there was a predictable increase in tension, with Mary fearing that Nan was "returning to her old ways" and Nan protesting that her mother was "constantly in my face." Resuming the task of calibrating their demands, the mother and daughter developed a pattern that brought both more freedom and more responsibility to Nan, in keeping with her age and the appropriate concerns of her mother.

The 2-year follow-up has been encouraging for the staff, as they consider the effects of the new approach. Nan has sustained her recovery, has held a steady job, and is planning to move into her own apartment. Mary and Janet have a companionable relationship, and the family reports that "we are all doing well."

The Case of Bud

Bud's case presented different issues. At 17, he was addicted to cocaine, was diagnosed as having attention-deficit/hyperactivity disorder (ADHD) and bipolar disorder, had a history of robberies, and was currently being offered one last chance by the courts. His family consisted of his mother and father, Karen and Martin, and two older siblings living on their own in different towns.

When the intake worker called the family and asked Karen to come in with Bud and her husband, Karen wasn't certain that Martin would be willing but said he would probably come, "at least to the first interview." Bud's father came and registered his resistance to being blamed for everything, but he agreed to work on positive solutions to the difficulties with Bud. The father had a strong personality, was prominent in the community, and was forceful in the family. In the screening interview, the worker saw a pattern emerging—mother and son in alliance against a strong father—but this first encounter focused on the need for the parents' cooperation and the sense of crisis concerning Bud.

In the next meeting, the tension was evident. Martin exploded in anger at Bud, Karen defended her son, Martin turned to lash out at Karen, and Bud said to his mother, "Why do you let him walk all over you?" The counselor relabeled Bud's problem as "immature and irresponsible behavior," rather than as "substance abuse," and that formulation became the guideline not only for the counselor but also for the house staff and the parole officer in their contacts with Bud. It was uncomfortable for the adolescent but a more hopeful formulation for the parents.

During the subsequent meetings, the pattern of attack, defense, coalition, and escalation became visible to all participants, and was recognized for its destructive effects. Now more alert to warning signs, the parents began to collaborate on setting rules. They decided, for instance, that when Bud came home, he would have to either work or go to college, and would need to pay for certain expenses.

On one of the first weekend visits, Bud challenged the rules. He borrowed the car without permission, and when Karen called the counselor she was asked, in a reminder of the new collaboration between the parents, "Did you talk with your husband about it?" Martin and Karen decided that the weekend visits would need to be suspended—a different-seeming consequence when the decision comes from the parents rather than the institution. Bud was angry, but in 2 weeks he called home and asked for a meeting. As with Nan and others, it was a turning point when the parents were able to exert firm control and the adolescent, first angry, then thoughtful, reached out to talk things over. In the next meeting, Bud admitted he was at fault, but he talked with his father about how upset he felt when Martin blew up and walked away instead of dealing with what was going on. "I need to change," said Bud, "but this is also everyone's problem in the family."

After this incident, the family became involved in catching the repetition of patterns on their own and looking for useful solutions. Bud commented, after one incident, "We solved it as a family, and that has never happened." As Bud moved to the reentry level, the family began to plan how they would organize family life and use the outreach program to maintain positive changes. For both the family and staff, it was remarkable that they had reached this point in 7 months, rather than the 18 months authorized for Bud's treatment program.

In this case, Bud's two-parent family suggested a focus different from the single-parent household and adult-partner structure that prevailed in Nan's case. A counselor begins with certain expectations of the forces that may be operating, simply because the adult–child system has particular features. During the family meetings, patterns specific to the family emerge, and the counselor works toward empowering the parents in a constructive way on the basis of their unique problems and potential strengths.

Sometimes, other family members are particularly important. In one case, for instance, the presence of a sibling was crucial. The alienation between the 18-year-old resident and his parents was rigid, but his 15-year-old brother, who had become his ally and was beginning to use drugs, provided a connecting link. The younger boy expressed both anger and a sense of abandonment, pleading for family change and offering the family counselor some leverage for working with this family. While the goals are always similar, the process of working with each family depends on its membership, structural patterns, and available sources of strength.

Changing Organizational Structures and Procedures

If a new approach is to be sustained, organizational structures and procedures must be modified. There were, in fact, widespread changes at the residence during the course of training. They were the result of extensive discussions at administrative meetings, which were held every 6 weeks, and at occasional retreats for the total staff. They reached into every corner of the enterprise: staff organization, screening and intake, the handling of decisions and crises, the activities of the Family Association, and collaboration with outside systems. The details are reviewed in the following section.

Revising Roles, Supervision, and In-House Training

The family approach was blocked, at first, by overload, confusing job descriptions, and a duplication of roles. As a result, the decision was made to draw firmer lines of responsibility between clinical workers and behavioral counselors. Clinical staff were now responsible for meeting with each family at least twice a month, while behavioral counselors were to manage in-house activities and monitor the behavior of the residents.

It had become clear that clinical workers needed more detailed supervision if they were to be effective, and the coordinator of family therapy began to meet weekly with this staff to review cases, observe tapes, and supervise live interviews. An in-house training structure was established, serving to orient new staff to the agency approach and providing more experienced personnel with the opportunity for further development. Supervisors continued to meet weekly with the consultant, bringing in difficult cases and issues of staff supervision for review.

Changing Staff Attitudes toward Families

At the final administrative meeting of the project, the consultant asked the nine assembled staff members, "What has changed, as a result of the training . . . and what has shifted to bring that about?" In responding to that question, staff members commented first on the shift in attitudes about the families. As one worker said:

> "We changed the way we think. When we started the training here, there were a lot of misgivings about how the family should be involved, because in the past the BCs [behavioral counselors] always had the say. We never used the resources of the family. . . . But once we started to mold our thinking, the family had to become more involved in regard to crises, in coming to sessions, in holding the kid accountable. I think a lot of us reshaped our thinking . . . and eventually, down the line, the staff bought into it."

That comment is a reminder that ideas and attitudes are the basis for workable procedural changes. It points also to individual differences in the pace of adaptation; it takes time for some staff members to "buy in." For the consultant, the statement signaled that the residence had moved beyond the mentality of a boarding school to that of a setting committed to temporary custody and a collaborative relationship with parents. The staff was no longer maintaining that "we are your family," and the change appeared, as well, in the mission statement of the residence, which had added the term "family based" to its description.

The Revision of Screening and the Intake Process

For the staff, the new process of screening and intake marked a fundamental change. They described the fact that now they start involving the family on "day one." They explain to the family that this residence is different from most centers; that staff members know they can't be helpful without the parents so they will be working with the family in a team effort. The new intake forms provide them with a framework for asking questions about relationships, and about people who might be helpful. The intake worker might ask, for instance, how Linda gets along with her younger brother, or whether the grandparents tend to stick up for Denzel when the parents are trying to lay down the law, or whether Samantha has a favorite aunt or uncle, or whether the parents are worried about drug use by other members of the family. And so forth.

The staff also uses the first meetings with a family to set up discharge objectives and arrive at agreements about how the adolescent's behavior must be different in order to return home.

Another major change, from the staff perspective, is the effort to know and understand the family from the beginning. "We map the system the way we were taught," one staff member says, "and the staff sometimes sees the information before they even meet the kid." Another comments:

> "We're joining with the family. It's not that we're the experts and we're going to make the rules and tell you how it's done . . . *they* are the experts. We've always concentrated on getting the kid to adjust to the residence, and that's important, but the ultimate goal is to get the kid to adjust to the home with the parents. . . . It's true that they have to do well here, but. . . ."

Including Parents in Decisions Concerning the Adolescent

Perhaps the most drastic change, from the perspective of a therapeutic model, is the participation of the parents in decisions and disciplinary procedures while the adolescent is in residence. Parents are now involved in the granting of privileges, the move to new levels, and questions of control and consequences. In a sense, the revisions have brought the parents into the executive structure, and, like the participants in the perinatal program, they have become stakeholders in this new approach.

Expanding the Family Association

The Family Association has become an important part of the structure, having grown in size and function, and the staff has been active in making that happen. When a family is screened, the worker emphasizes both a commitment to family therapy and an involvement in the Family Association. A staff member says:

> "We've gotten better at getting families to come to the Family Association. We tie going home to Family Association participation. You want your kid to come home. We want him to come home too, but if you're not coming to the Family Association, we're gonna hold back on that until you come . . . because we need you to be ready to receive him. To put it another way, we need you to be a more effective parent, and you can learn to be a more effective parent by going to the Family Association."

The Family Association has also become more active in contacting new applicants. The staff explains that, for the past 2 years, when intake is finished, the information is transferred to the chairman of the Welcome Committee, and the membership reaches out and makes a personal connection, inviting the family to participate in the association. It gives the family a person and phone number they can call if they have a question, and it gets them involved right away—sometimes even before their adolescent has a place at the residence.

In the current structure, parents attend meetings both of the Family Association and of the newly formed Multiple Family Groups. A staff member explains the difference: "Well, the kids are part of the Multiple Family sessions, and the emphasis is a lot more on the transition of the parents having the kid back, after all these months. They walk on eggshells, so to speak. And there's the transition for the kid also, in being home and getting to see what's different." These sessions are also helpful when the youngsters have earned home visits and issues arise that need to be discussed with others who have gone through the same experience. The Family Association meetings, on the other hand, are only for parents. As one staff member said, "It's more a peer-to-peer identification. In some cases, the families are quite broken, and they need to put that together again."

Modifying Contacts with Courts, Schools, and Aftercare Programs

Families are now included in staff liaisons with the courts, the probation system, the schools, and aftercare. The probation system now works with both the adolescent and the family, and aftercare programs include family in the continuum of care during transitions between the residence and outpatient facilities. In keeping with the new understanding of what a family faces when the adolescent comes home, there's an increased focus on this vulnerable period, as well as a shift from the philosophy of crisis intervention to one of prevention and ongoing support.

Staff Recruitment and Functioning

New structures and formal procedures are often easier to maintain, once they are established, than the daily implementation of a new approach by staff members. The work required to help an adolescent adapt to the residence is demanding, and it's difficult to focus on the family at the same time. Staff turnover also tends to bring slippage in the new ways of working. As one person remarked, "When there's turnover, there's a step back. . . .We need to be conscious of that."

The administrators see staff functioning as an area of necessary vigilance, and are focusing not only on supervision and in-house training but also on recruitment policies. When administrators interview people for clinical positions, they require a degree or certification and are trying to elevate the requirements. They explain that they are looking for people who understand the behavioral work of the community but are trained in family therapy, and they regard that as a big organizational change.

Extending the Family Focus to a New Site

When the organization began construction of a new facility, planning included a family orientation from the beginning. Training in family work began as soon as the first new staff members were hired, and adolescents who would be the first clients were bussed to the site every 3 weeks for a family day.

The training situation for the new consultant was very different

from that at the original facility.[5] Here, the organization was fully committed to working with families, but the situation was in flux. Staff
members were hired slowly, they varied considerably in their experience and familiarity with family work, and they had no history of
working together. A trainer who is beginning to teach in such a situation has both advantages and problems. The integration of a family
orientation into structures and procedures means, in effect, that it is
part of the job description when new staff sign on, and that is an advantage. Whatever their confusion or resistance, newcomers know they
will be expected to work in this way and that the training is relevant for
the skills they will need. On the other hand, the slow accumulation of
staff and the wide variety of their past experiences means that the logical progression in the training program cannot register with all staff
members in the same way. In spite of that reality, the trainer must follow an organized sequence of teaching, and must problem solve, along
with the administrative staff, as difficulties arise.

The consultant began with an overview of system concepts, family
organization, techniques for assessment, mapping, and first sessions
with a family, followed by the presentation of videotapes and demonstration interviews. The latter were used as springboards for discussions of joining, enactment, reframing, complementarity, the search for
family strength, and so forth. In general, that "curriculum" is typical of
trainers with the viewpoint we have been describing.

New staff members who missed this orientation were frequently
stymied by the discrepancy between family-oriented procedures and
the principles that had guided their previous work. As a result, the
director of family work assumed the task of orienting new staff concerning the basic ideas before they joined the training group. In addition, those staff members who were already established assured the
newcomers that these strange ideas would become clearer over time.
In reassuring others, of course, they were also cementing their own
learning and their commitment to a family focus. By the end of the
first year, the staff had learned something about working with families, particularly if they had participated in the training from the
beginning. They had become relatively comfortable in family ses-

---

[5]Daniel Minuchin, MA, the consultant/trainer at this site, contributed the material for this section.

sions, had developed some skills, and were showing their videotapes for supervision and discussion.

The situation at the new residence remains a work in progress. As the program moved into the second year, the residence filled with adolescents, and personnel faced the necessity of putting ideas into practice. The staff would be implementing the program, working out the balance between the activities of the therapeutic community and the involvement of parents, handling crises, counseling families, and fine-tuning the responsibilities and boundaries of each staff member's role. For their part, administrators and supervisors would be focused on maintaining the policies and procedures that establish a family-oriented program. They would also be working to achieve the integrated structure and prevailing sense of accomplishment that characterizes the residence that pioneered this program.

WHAT ENABLES A NEW APPROACH TO SURVIVE?

The introduction of a family perspective into drug treatment centers, combined with the subsequent history of developments, has taught us something about how interventions survive; what makes them effective during the training and capable of continuation afterward. In this final section of the chapter, we discuss six factors that have supported the survival of family practices in these settings, four that emerged in connection with both programs and two with particular relevance for one situation or the other.

The four factors that apply to both programs are as follows:

- Integration into organizational policies and procedures.
- Leadership commitment.
- The creation and involvement of stakeholders.
- Adaptability.

The following factor was important for the residential center for adolescents:

- Intensive family-oriented training and supervision.

The following factor was important for the perinatal program:

- The support of social policies.

Integration into Organizational Policies and Procedures

For proponents of a new approach, the disappearance of effects they have helped to create is profoundly disappointing. Often the training goes well and research confirms the impression that things have changed, but when the trainers move on, the waters close over what has been built. Perhaps the most effective protection against the force of erosion is the integration of new policies and procedures into the ongoing work of the institution.

That process was particularly clear at the residence for adolescents, where the relatively independent structure allowed the firm adoption of new procedures. In the end, family intake, counseling, and decision making were simply an expression of how this residence worked, along with supervision of the staff's work with families, a central role for the Family Association, and family-oriented contacts with external systems. Though the adolescent center functioned within a more dependable context than most public services can expect, it provides a useful example of the process through which a new approach becomes an integral part of the institution.

The situation for the perinatal project was probably closer to the realities of most public services; decisions elsewhere in the system can always jeopardize new procedures. Yet it was possible to maintain basic elements of the program through integration into a permanent hospital department. Within that structure, there was space and support for family-oriented activities that had begun and developed elsewhere. The continuation of multidisciplinary case conferences at the Ob/Gyn Department further strengthened the family focus, since it involved personnel from other parts of the hospital who had become interested in the orientation and adopted that framework in their contacts with the women.

Leadership Commitment

Most interventions start with enthusiasm on both sides but it becomes difficult to maintain energy and commitment over time. Consultants are discouraged by resistance and recurrent obstacles; administrators find that requirements for new procedures interfere with the smooth operation of their agency. A new approach can only be consolidated, however, if the commitment of key personnel is maintained.

The programs described in this chapter would have foundered

without the sustained efforts of the people in leadership positions—both the teams that introduced the interventions and the administrators at the institutions. The consultant/trainer of the perinatal project continued his work when the venue changed, even through periods when previous gains were lost and financial support disappeared. The counterpart for his leadership came from the director and staff of the hospital department. They provided a strong commitment to core elements of the program and a necessary base for family-oriented activities.

The task for leaders at the residential center was less stressful but equally essential. The administrator who had initiated the program steered the agency through periods of uncertainty, working with the staff and the consultant so that the new approach would fit comfortably into the style and purpose of the agency. The commitment of the consultant included both immediate and long-term goals. He was involved in staff training from the beginning, but he focused as well on helping the agency develop mechanisms for resolving its own issues, so that it could maintain a family orientation and function effectively after he left.

The Creation and Involvement of Stakeholders

When a new approach is introduced, a major goal is to change the thinking and practice of administrators and staff; in other words, to consult and train personnel so effectively that they become stakeholders in this way of working, prepared to carry it forward. That may be obvious. What is less obvious is that the intervention is, or should be, aimed at creating stakeholders among the clients; participants who experience the benefits of the program and are invested in its continuation. In both drug treatment settings, we witnessed the creation and involvement of family-oriented stakeholders among the recipients of service.

As these two programs suggest, the primary stakeholders in a situation are not always the identified clients. The perinatal women would clearly be the stakeholders in the first program, but the potential stakeholders in the second program were actually the parents. At the beginning of these projects, neither the perinatal women nor the parents saw themselves as forces in shaping the process of treatment—the pregnant women because they were accustomed to a relatively powerless position in public service systems and the parents because their children were the focus of professional efforts. A primary purpose in both projects, however, was to bring these groups to center stage, helping them to develop a sense of involvement and self-direction. In retrospect, it seems clear that the evolution of involved and self-directed stakeholders was a factor in supporting the survival of a family approach.

The process took time and went through stages. The perinatal women were initially brought into family-oriented groups that were set up and run by staff. Parents of the adolescents were first called in to participate in admissions procedures, then consulted on decisions concerning their children. Gradually, as these experiences were repeated, the pregnant women and the parents became more active and independent. The perinatal women began to run their own groups, made decisions about who could come to the clinic to support them, and reached out into the community to contact others in their situation. At the adolescent center, a token association of parents became a large and active organization, offering help to new parents, establishing family groups in the community, and meeting to discuss the issues of transition, relapse, and aftercare.

It's important to note that both "involvement" and "self-direction" are necessary aspects of this role, and that they are likely to develop sequentially. Clients are often used to being in the role of recipients. A staff that wants to facilitate the creation of stakeholders must first help the group to become involved, then cede power for making meaningful decisions and solving problems. In both programs, the trainers and staff first organized participant activities, then left direction to the group members as the latter signaled that they had become more confident and knowledgeable.

Adaptability

The need for realistic and flexible adaptability applies both to the proponents of a new approach and to the institution that has requested training. It begins with the first contact between the team of trainers and the agency and involves what we generally refer to as "joining." That is, the consultants must respect the agency's evaluation of what they want and need, even as they make their own evaluation of the organization and consider the implications for their project. As time goes on, some adaptations are inevitable, but it's important to be aware of the difference between elements of the model that are so essential they cannot be sacrificed and elements that can be modified without significant damage.

The most dramatic challenge to the family orientation in either setting came from the official termination of the perinatal program.

The combination of forces that enabled continuation, including both the acceptance of the inevitable and the search for solutions, offers an impressive example of resilience and adaptation. The residential center faced no comparable threat to the survival of the new approach, but the need for flexibility became evident when the program expanded to a new setting, where circumstances were different and routines were less established.

If adaptability is a necessary ingredient for the survival of a model over time, questions must be raised about models that are deliberately self-contained—that prepare their staff to adhere closely to training manuals, have specific requirements for participants, and are evaluated through tightly controlled research. These models, as well as the accompanying research, have been invaluable for putting concepts and practices into the field, but, as Rowe and Liddle (2003) have noted, they have not transferred well to communities and public services, which operate in the midst of ever-changing realities and cannot guarantee specific conditions for more than short periods. To be broadly effective, these models would need to become more flexible, searching for the balance between maintaining the most essential standards and adapting to the complexities of system realities.

Intensive Family-Oriented Training and Supervision

The importance of this factor emerged at the residential center. It was not relevant for the therapeutic community, which expected the outside team to conduct family work with the perinatal clients and did not request training for its staff. The residential center, however, was seeking training that would enable their staff to work effectively with families. From that experience, it appears that the establishment of changes that will endure depends on two things: the nature and duration of the training program itself, and the possibility of continuing supervision and review within the institution after the program has finished.

The training program itself was intensive, involving a baseline of theory, experiential activities, demonstrations by experienced teachers, and supervised work with families. In addition, the consultant worked with the staff on solving institutional problems by drawing on their own resources. Such matters take time. The program lasted for three years, and the extended contact between the trainer and the staff was an important element in the success of the program.

Even with extended training, the danger that new ways of working will go down in quality or disappear over time is very real; newly minted family counselors are often discouraged in the face of difficult situations, and staff turnover brings in workers who have not shared the earlier training. The establishment of structures within the residential center for continuing review and development has provided an important safeguard, serving to control slippage and sustain the effects of the training. In effect, the training continues in-house, though the form and content of this institutional phase is different from the intensive program.

The Support of Social Policies

This factor came to the fore in relation to the perinatal program, and was relevant mostly in consideration of policies that do not support a family orientation. There are many ways of defining policies that support families, of course, but for our work the most relevant are those that apply to the delivery of services, especially, though not exclusively, for the less advantaged portions of society. Over the last 40 years or so, the nation has gone through different phases in its concern for poor families, having featured a variety of supportive policies during the War on Poverty and shifting over time to a perspective that is more focused on the individual and less concerned with this population.

The factor of social support will become important again at the end of the book when we review what we have learned from all the interventions. We identify this factor now, however, because the perinatal program provided an interesting insight: The program could continue on the basis of other factors we have described as long as social policies did not actively interfere with family-oriented procedures. Once an official mandate required particular conditions of residence for substance-dependent pregnant women, however, it became impossible for families to meet at the hospital department, and the program was curtailed. What emerges for discussion, from this example, is not so much the value of social, theoretical, and economic supports for a family approach—which, from our point of view, can hardly be questioned—but the consideration of how to persist when the social atmosphere is not supportive. In troubled times, that question is at the heart of interventions concerned with people who have little power.

CHAPTER SIX

Foster Care
Children, Families, and the System

Despite changes in the conception of viable family structures in recent decades, our understanding of what children require for healthy development remains the same: security, nurturance, social contacts, and guidance. Each family manages these functions in their own way, but society has set limits on what is considered an acceptable environment for children and has established procedures for removing them from home if the standards are not met. In these early years of the 21st century, we have more than half a million children in foster care across the nation (Marx, Benoit, & Kamradt, 2003). It is a startling figure. Why are there so many? Is foster care the best alternative in all of these cases? And is it possible to improve the process of evaluation, placement, and continuing service so that children and families can progress effectively toward a more functional future?

In the view of mental health professionals who have surveyed the foster care population, children in foster care are among the most disturbed young people in the country (Marx et al., 2003). They suggest that the children have been severely damaged by their early experiences and that the situation can best be remedied by changing the context and providing extensive psychological services. On closer inspection, however, that view appears limited. Focused primarily on history and treatment, it does not take into account the process of removal, placement, and adaptation when children are taken into care or ponder the effects of that experience.

It's surprising that a profession which considers attachment to be the basis for security and healthy growth does not highlight the potential for anxiety when children are uprooted from familiar settings. The young are generally attached to the people they have known, even if the adults have been neglectful or inconsistent, and even if the children are offered a new situation that is potentially more supportive. A carefully considered separation may be useful, at least temporarily, and when there is actual abuse, removal is necessary. But the process itself is inevitably traumatic, affecting the adaptation of both children and families.

Our approach is systemic. We see the foster care experience as a complex combination of children, families, and service systems, and we consider the impact on the children before, during, and after placement. From that broader view, we are slower to decide why these children are so troubled, less certain that removal from their families is the best solution in all cases, and more focused on possibilities for improving the foster care system at various points in the process and at various levels of the network surrounding the children.

In this chapter, we describe a systemic approach to foster care, formulated and implemented over a period of more than 20 years. The chapter is divided into two sections, reporting two blocks of work that are connected but separate. They share a systemic orientation and a concern with the same population of multicrisis clients, but changes in official policies over time have brought new issues to the fore and the second program has necessarily focused on different aspects of the foster care experience. Together, the two programs offer a breadth of detail about working within the system.

In the first section, we present the basic principles of a systemic, or "ecological," model, highlighting the central triangle of biological family, foster family, and professional workers, and describing the concepts that are essential to the well-being of all participants. We then describe the implementation of the model through a training project of several years with foster care agencies: the communication of new ideas, the facilitation of new skills for staff, the effort to change agency policies and procedures, and the direct work with families to help them become more viable settings for the growth of their children. This work was conducted by the staffs of Family Studies, Inc. and the Minuchin Center for the Family.[1]

In the second section, we present the Foster Care Project developed by Jorge Colapinto. This work deals with the increasing recognition of "child time" as an important factor in the foster care experience and with the necessity for permanency planning on behalf of the child. The project has addressed the elements of delay and fragmentation in the system that dilute effective functioning and leave the children adrift. In the process, the staff has developed concrete materials and behavioral tools for facilitating the effectiveness of procedures and decisions.

In the first project, we were working within foster care agencies, training staff and collaborative teams to work effectively with families. In the second project, the emphasis was on the system, and on the blockage that jeopardizes a successful resolution for the child. We see these projects as complementary. Foster care involves a complex system and a sustained process. To create effective change, it's essential to intervene at multiple levels and at different points of the process.

AN ECOLOGICAL MODEL:
CONCEPTS AND IMPLEMENTATION

The stated aims of foster care have often reflected a compassionate philosophy, highlighting the goals of relieving stress in overburdened families, caring for their children during an interim period, and increasing their ability to care safely for the young so the family can be reunited. In practice, however, the process of evaluation, placement, and continuing service has often defeated these aims, and our work has focused on bringing foster care practice closer to the original goals.

The approach to foster care, as described in this chapter, was developed by Salvador Minuchin (1984). Based on general concepts about families and systems, the model was adapted to the specific realities of the foster care situation and subsequently applied to staff

---

[1]Staff involved in different phases of the project included Salvador Minuchin, Director, and Evan Bellin, Anne Brooks, Jorge Colapinto, Ema Genijovich, Daniel Minuchin, and Patricia Minuchin.

training in foster care agencies. The aim has been to reduce trauma, build family strength, and increase the possibility of successful reunification. In order to achieve these goals, the model has emphasized connections among parts of the system, empowerment of the child's family, and the expansion of roles for both professional staff and members of the foster and biological families. The model is unique, but the aims have been shared by other family-oriented organizations. The Annie E. Casey Foundation, for example, has been supporting the broad Family to Family Initiative since the 1990s (DeMuro & Rideout, 2002; Sharkey, 1997; Thielman, 2001).

In presenting this project, we will describe the basic concepts of what we have come to call the "ecological model," followed by the details of training and consultation in foster care agencies. We begin, however, with a brief review of the foster care system in the large metropolitan area within which we were working: the involvement of municipal departments, courts, and foster care agencies, and the process that went from the first complaints through placement and subsequent procedures. Though the details describe the particular context within which we first implemented the model, they are characteristic of the foster care system in many areas, and they point to the aspects of the process that require attention and revision.

The Context: Larger Systems and the Process of Placement

The process usually begins when protective services are informed that a child is being abused or neglected. An investigator may decide that there is no basis for the allegation or that the situation can be handled by direct services to the family, but in many cases the decision is made that the child must be removed from the home. Sometimes that decision is obviously correct; in other cases, it is questionable, reflecting limited information, the evaluation of a poverty-stricken household as necessarily a negative environment for children, or fear of criticism if the child remains and is harmed. When tragic cases come to public attention, workers feel a new urgency in the unofficial mandate "When in doubt, remove the child."

After removal, the child is placed with an accredited foster family, and court hearings set the terms of reunification. The plan may call for some combination of parenting classes, personal counseling, drug treatment, anger management, and so forth. At intervals, the courts will review progress, as reported by protective services and

agency workers. During the period of placement, visiting arrangements depend on the agency, but visits are typically scheduled once
every two weeks on agency premises. The child's family has little
power during the removal and court hearings, and when the child is
placed in foster care, contact between biological and foster families is
usually minimal or nonexistent.

The intention is a protective one, but judgmental attitudes, limited understanding of family connections, and bureaucratic fragmentation of services tend to create a situation of drift. The child's relatives begin to miss visits, and the child and foster family bond while
child and biological parents become increasingly detached. If family
reunification occurs at some later point, it is often unsuccessful. In
creating a different model, we were concerned with changing both
the guiding ideas that shaped this system and the practical procedures.

The Ecological Model: Six Basic Ideas

Foster care has unique features. Unlike most social services, foster
placement involves two families: the biological family and the foster
family. There are also two sets of agency "employees": the professional staff and the foster families. With this reality in mind, we formulated six basic ideas as the core of the ecological model.

Foster Placement Creates a New, Triangular System

As soon as a child is separated from home and placed in a foster family, a new triangular system comes into being. It is composed of the
biological family, the foster family, and the foster care agency, all of
which are connected inevitably by their concern for the same child.
That reality is not often acknowledged within the foster care system.
Indeed, the usual procedures tend to create a sharp demarcation
between the two families, and the fragmentation of services often
means that professional workers miss the connections.

Within that triangular network, there are important subsystems:
the unit of foster and biological families, the team of social worker
and foster family, and the child within the context of each family—a
participant in the patterns of both. From the perspective of this
model, the existence of a superordinate triangle, and of subsystems
within it, is a basic fact.

The Triangular System Should Be Collaborative Rather Than Adversarial, and Should Include the Members of Both Families

If the first idea is a description of reality, the second is a statement of goals—perhaps the core of the approach. If policymakers and professional workers could think in these terms and organize procedures accordingly, the foster care system would be on its way to improving the experience and the probable outcome (see P. Minuchin, 1995).

Collaboration implies that people are in contact with each other and that they function as a network, sharing information and solving problems by mutual effort. In the typical foster care situation, members of the triangular system are rarely in that kind of contact. Professional work is often limited to the one adult in each family who seems primarily responsible for the child—usually the biological or foster mother. Workers seldom search for members of the extended biological family who might be a resource even if they don't live with mother and child, and they rarely make contact with all the members of the foster household, though they will all affect how the new child is received.

When members of the two families meet, typically during visits between mother and child at the agency, the contact is usually brief and the tone wary or adversarial. Foster and biological families tend to view each other stereotypically, and their attitudes are often negative. When Roger and Alva Lincoln took Jed into their home as a foster child, they were told only that he had been neglected by his parents, and they wondered aloud how anybody "could do that to a child." Jed's mother and father were bewildered by the speed with which Jed and his sister were removed from the family, and they resented the people "who've got our kids." As with all stereotypes, these attitudes are not easily altered, especially without contact between families.

The quality of contact between members of the two families is at the heart of the matter, and has much to do with the eventual outcome. Kelsey's case is useful to consider, since she has participated both in a destructive relationship and one that is sustained and supportive.

Kelsey left home at 13 with a man in his 20s who was drug addicted. She left him after the birth of her second child. She is now 17 and her sons are both in foster care, but they have been placed in separate homes monitored by different agencies. Kelsey has tried to maintain contact with both children but has had very different experiences with the two foster families.

Kelsey talks first about her contacts with the foster mother of her younger son during visits with the boy at the agency:

> "She brings him in when she wants to bring him. Like, if I have a visit from 12 to 4, she'll bring him in at 3:30. . . . She tells me, 'Don't pick him up. Don't kiss him. Don't take him outside.' So I say he's my son, and she says, 'Yeah, well he's in my care now, so he's my son.' And I'll be crying, but nobody does nothing about it. So I just gave up. When I get my son, I'll just take him and go!"

The downward spiral is obvious. The combination of Kelsey's complaints, the criticisms of the foster mother, and the fact that Kelsey no longer visits her son will probably lead the agency to consider her a surly, irresponsible mother who's not interested in the child. Her assumption that she will one day get her son back and can "just go" is naive, and her expectation that things will be all right when that time comes is doubly so. It's unlikely that she will function well as a parent, if she were suddenly to assume that role with an uprooted, bewildered young child who knows her less well than he knows the foster family.

Kelsey's experience with the foster family of her 3-year-old is different. Kelsey and the foster mother have established a strong relationship. "Julie's cool," says Kelsey.

> "When I first came here, I had a nasty attitude. I didn't want to talk to nobody . . . 'cause they had my son! I'd complain about everything: 'I don't like this; I don't like that. Why has he got a scratch on him?'—knowing he's gonna fall . . . knowing when I had him he'd fall. But I'd go on about anything, just to get mad. . . . And Julie, she'd come over to me and say, 'Kelsey, you know boys! Come on now, whyn't you stop that?' And she'd talk to me, and I'd still be . . . like 'grrrrr' . . . and she'd say, 'Well look, let's take Buddy and go get some lunch.' "

Starting with the same anger she felt when each son was taken away, Kelsey responds to warmth, humor, and the matter-of-fact

acceptance of her resentment. She also profits from the small, effective ways the foster mother makes space for her relationship with her
son, encouraging Kelsey's competence and providing a model for
handling the concrete tasks of socializing a young child. Kelsey says:

> "You know, sometimes Buddy'll ask Julie something and she'll
> say, 'Whyn't you go ask Mommy to take your jacket off . . . or
> ask Mommy to take you to the bathroom?' Things I didn't
> know, I wasn't embarrassed to ask her. She potty trained him,
> and she'd be telling me things . . . so I asked her, 'How did you
> get Buddy to do that? And how do you get Buddy to go to bed at
> a certain time?', 'cause with me, if he don't want to go to bed, I
> won't make him go to bed. So, she was saying you have to let
> him know you're the mother and it's time to go to bed. And
> sometimes Buddy'll get mad at me, and he'll say, 'I hate you!',
> and I ask her how am I supposed to deal with that? I ask her
> things and she tells me how she does with him, so when he
> comes home I can do the same."

The difference in these two experiences is not just a matter of the
personality of the foster parent. It's a function of the preparation of
the foster family, in terms of understanding, compassion, and skills,
and of the agency policies and supports that make this kind of contact possible.

Empowerment of the Biological Family Is Crucial

A collaborative network, in the foster care situation, depends on reasonable equality in the roles of its members. When a child is taken
for placement, the biological family is at the low point of the triangle. Society has established a hierarchy of approval: the foster family
is competent and the biological family inadequate. If parents are to
manage the period of placement and the possibility of reunification
successfully, they must regain the sense that they have some role in
relation to the lives of their children.

Consider the experience of Nelda. She has four children: a 19-
year-old son who has a steady job and lives on his own, and three
children who live with her. Tommy, 14, attends school; Rafie, 4, is
mildly mentally handicapped; and Damon, a sickly infant, is failing
to thrive. When Nelda takes the baby to the hospital, the nurse is

alarmed and alerts protective services. A worker sent to inspect the home reports garbage bags standing in the kitchen, little food in the refrigerator, and a general atmosphere of squalor and disarray. She returns the next day with a police officer and they remove the three children, leaving a distraught and bewildered mother with an explanation that it's for the good of the baby and that she will be notified of a court hearing. The children are placed according to their needs and available venues: the infant in a city hospital, the 4-year-old with a suburban family accredited for the special care of mentally handicapped children, and the 14-year-old in a distant institution for adolescents separated from home. The geography of these placements is daunting. How can the mother keep contact with all the children?

At the hearing, there's no provision for Nelda to speak for herself. She wants to explain that the garbage bags were waiting for her 19-year-old son to carry them down; that she was going shopping for food that afternoon; that her sister sometimes takes the children while she cleans her house. She wants to explain how she copes, and the fact that nobody in power will listen leaves her angry and depressed.

The plan for reunification involves parenting classes, personal counseling, and regular visits with the children. If these are the conditions, she's more than willing and follows the plan. However, when interviewed by a person she trusts, Nelda admits feeling confused and hopeless. Traveling to visit the children is exhausting, and the parenting classes seem irrelevant. Most of all, she's bewildered by the counseling. Nobody has explained what's wrong, what's expected of her, or how she will know when her actions are successful. People who trudge through a prescription in this way feel powerless; it's unlikely that Nelda will be more competent or confident when and if her children are returned.

The process could be different. The fact that Nelda has raised her two older boys successfully should be part of the equation. It was probably unnecessary to remove the 14-year-old, who was attending school and well behaved, and the placement of the two younger boys could have been handled in a way that made the mother a partner, preparing her through a personalized program to care effectively for children with problems. Rather than attending general parenting classes, she would have profited from contact with the hospital staff concerning her sickly infant, and with the specialized foster mother concerning the education of her mentally challenged youngster.

The problems in this case centered on the nature of the placements and the fact that mandated activities were not oriented to the realities of this family. In other cases, the problems arise from agency procedures, which organize intake and visitation in ways that underscore the biological family's lack of power, even when that is not the intent. It is possible, however, to convey a different, more positive message.

Consider the following situation: Two small boys have been placed with a foster family and the parents have not seen them for 3 months. A trainer has been working with the agency responsible for the case, and the social worker arranges for the parents to come in for a meeting with the two children and the foster parents.

As they all settle down, the foster mother puts the 1-year-old on her lap and reaches for a diaper. The social worker suggests that the child's mother can do that. The foster mother is willing and hands the child over; it just didn't occur to her. The social worker, alert to the importance of communication between these two families, suggests that the foster parents describe their family so that the other couple can picture the new setting for their children. As the foster parents talk about their children, telling the couple that the 6-year-old is a special pal for their two boys, the conversation becomes friendly and tension is reduced. At the same time, it becomes obvious that the foster family has been calling the older boy "Kenny," the name on his official records, although he has been called "Kiko" by his family since birth—and that he has been slow to respond. Furthermore, "We didn't know he could walk till last week, when he got up and ran across the room after the dog!" Even though they did not say so, this family had clearly been treating the 2-year-old as a child with mental retardation, slow to walk, talk, and recognize his name.

The trainer remarked that the child must have been very frightened by the changes in his life and began to talk with the mother about Kiko's development: When did he first sit up? What words can he say? As the mother responded with details, the trainer commented that the parents really did know a lot about the children's early life that the foster parents don't know, and all agreed. The families were now on the verge of forming an alliance in which all could be seen as contributors.

In that situation, the trainer and the social worker were the motors of change, encouraging interaction between the two families. However, our training project also prepared foster parents to relate in a constructive way with the parents of the children they had in care, and they often generated effective ideas on their own. In the following example, a group of foster mothers were discussing the challenge of involving mothers in the care of their infants during visits. Knowing that the babies were bonded to the foster parent and that their birth mothers did not feel securely connected to the children, they had concrete suggestions for how to handle the problem. Martha says:

> "Right away I give the mother the baby, a bottle, some food, a Pamper. Now it's her baby. I don't tell her that, but . . . I may stay with her a little while and chat, but I always move away."

Gina nods, and adds:

> "I do the same thing. Maybe I go to the bathroom . . . and I'll stand outside the door about 10 or 15 minutes, because to me the mother . . . this is strange to her now, when she gets the baby in her hands, so I just let her know . . . 'Oh, the baby's hair needs to be combed. Could you comb her hair? I'll be right back. And could you change the Pamper for the baby? I got to go to the bathroom.' Not saying I want her to be able to . . . but she's got to know she's the mother. Not only that, but the baby has to know that's somebody in her life!"

Empowering biological families is both humane and psychologically sound. Only a family that feels respected and has some control over their own lives can provide a more functional environment for their children.

Major Transitions in Foster Care Require Special Attention

Foster care involves profound transitions, from removal and placement through all the subsequent moves. These are periods of upheaval, and the handling of the process shapes the course of future events.

In our training, we emphasize the challenge of the transition for everybody—not only the child, whose behavior may reflect the trauma of separation and the strangeness of the new situation, but also the foster and biological families. When a 5-year-old enters a foster home, everything changes—the way the adults function, how the siblings relate to each other, and how the routines of daily life are carried out. The biological family faces different but equally demanding issues. They must adapt to life without the children and must fulfill the various mandates that are prerequisites for reunification. Hostility or withdrawal are not surprising first reactions, and, as in the case of the children, may reflect the trauma of the separation rather than a confirmed attitude. Kelsey's comments described her "attitude" when the children were taken, and the process through which it changed.

Visits during placement are also small transitions, and the burden falls mostly on the child. We describe this with a concrete image (see Figure 6.1). The child is moving from one family to the other and back again, carrying a backpack. The backpack contains the expectations and patterns of the biological family, which the child carries into the foster family, as well as the expectations and patterns of the foster family, which are carried back on visits home. The child must fit into the patterns of each family, shifting with every move and integrating the mixture, somehow, into an internal map of the family world.

If the family is eventually reunited, the transition is welcome but not simple. It involves loss for the foster family and a challenge for the biological family, which must create a viable situation despite a history of adjudged failure. The task is realistically difficult. During

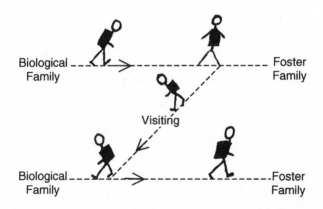

FIGURE 6.1. Visiting during foster care placement.

the period of placement, these parents and children have not experienced the kind of daily contact through which most of us work out relationships, set family rules, and establish credibility with each other.

More often than not, children return to a situation that is different from the one they left. They have changed, and so have their families. An 11-year-old whose destructive behavior has improved after 2 years returns to a family where there are new issues concerning a cousin suspected of molesting the older sister. Or a 4-year-old returns to a mother who has a new partner and another child. Reunification is a mixture of pleasure and discomfort. The transition requires careful planning, an understanding that successful adaptations take time, and a commitment by staff to continue their work until the situation has stabilized.

A Consideration of Developmental Issues Must Be Integrated into Foster Care Services

The child's stage of development shapes every aspect of the foster care experience, including the impact of separation, the adaptation to a new home, and the possibility of maintaining a sense of the original family while accepting new people. The reality is not necessarily easier or harder for children of different ages, but it's processed by different levels of understanding and emotion.

We know that different psychological issues come to the fore as children grow older. For infants, the basic issue is attachment: the child's sense of security invested in particular people and the adult sense of emotional investment in this child. When mothers and infants are separated early, basic attachment is jeopardized. Elena, for instance, has been hospitalized for a year and her baby has bonded to the foster mother. When Elena picks him up during visits, he cries and reaches for the foster mother. If Elena and her child are ever to live together, the foster mother must encourage their connection, and the social worker must help Elena with her deep sense of discouragement.

For toddlers and preschool children, as well as the adults who take care of them, the challenge is to find a balance between autonomy and control; between opportunities to explore the environment and the acceptance of realistic limits. Kelsey had little experience or skill in raising a young child: for getting her son to go to bed, for potty training, or for knowing when to accept the assertiveness of a 3-year-old and when to draw the line. With the help of the foster mother, she was learning firmness, patience, and judgment.

With children in their middle years, developmental issues arise in the family and in relation to school. Children of eight or nine have both privileges and responsibilities in a household. Families handle these differently, and a foster child carries both models in his or her "backpack." Sometimes the mixture of expectations creates a burden for the child. Mary's biological mother, for example, wanted her 10-year-old daughter to attend church regularly, but their Pentecostal church wasn't a comfortable choice for the foster parents. To relieve Mary's confusion, the adults discussed their dilemma and found a solution. The exchange of ideas for this situation created a pattern for handling other issues as well, particularly in regard to Mary's progress and comfort in the new school. Arrangements were made for her mother to attend parent meetings, and she met periodically with the foster parents to discuss how the child was adapting.

The developmental issues of adolescents are familiar and daunting: the need to move away from family while staying connected; the pull of the peer group; the pressure for individual decisions concerning drugs, sex, school, and future; the reality, for some, of violence in the community. Adolescents are often taken from their family because the adults can't control them. Helping a family qualify for reunification is more than a matter of drug programs, individual counseling, or skill training for parents and adolescents. They must develop a viable way of living together. It's neither correct nor productive for the foster family to work on developmental issues without involving the biological family, and it's unrealistic to expect the family to reunite successfully if they have been out of contact.

Kinship Care Creates a Unique Foster Care Situation

Most aspects of the ecological model apply to all foster care situations, but kinship care is different in one crucial way: When children are placed with relatives, the placement does not create a new system. Rather, it changes the reality of family members who already know each other and have established patterns of relating, carrying authority, and resolving conflict.

Kinship care is generally the preferred form of placement since it has clear psychological advantages for the child. It reduces the trauma of separation and does not require adaptation to a new world of people and places. Placing a child with familiar kin also increases the possibility that the "foster family" will continue to figure in the child's life and will function as a resource when the child returns home.

But kinship placements are not always simple. The extended family may be part of the problem as well as part of the solution. Arna's grandmother, for example, has long disapproved of her daughter's companions and way of life, and when she has the child in her care, she makes it difficult for mother and child to visit with each other. She argues over the visiting schedule, criticizes her daughter's way of handling Arna, and uses the opportunity to point out again that her daughter's friends are ruining her life. In other situations, relations are close but system boundaries are confused. If placement and reunification are to succeed, such issues must be identified and resolved, and the most constructive interventions are likely to be closer to conventional family therapy than is typical with foster care cases.

The family of Jill and her 3-year-old daughter, Margo, offers an illustration. Margo was in foster care, and her home visits were always spent at her grandmother's house. Jill would join her there so they could spend time together. When the social worker began to discuss family reunification, it became clear that Jill and her mother had different expectations. Jill saw them as "one big family." She expected Margo to move from the foster home to her grandmother's house, where she could visit her often. Jill commented that she had left her mother's home long ago but "not in my heart." The grandmother was startled: "I thought when you left home, you left home!" With three other children and serious economic problems, she had not expected to function as Margo's permanent caretaker, albeit unofficially.

The brief and successful course of therapy centered first on Jill and her mother, exploring Jill's immature expectations and the burden they placed on her mother. As that became clear, Jill's boyfriend joined the sessions. Together with the social worker, he and Jill discussed Margo's return to Jill's home, how that would affect the relationship of the couple, and what role he would play in the transition. The grandmother was now an interested but peripheral observer, and, after some sessions, the young couple continued without her. Despite the foster care context, family therapists would recognize this as a familiar situation, in which parents and young adult children must clarify boundaries and move toward a new stage of family equilibrium.

Training in Foster Care Settings

How to get from here to there? A model provides the ideas that shape values and goals, but the training process is a separate matter. It requires a theory about creating change and a sequential plan, as well as an awareness of the complexity of the task. Foster care agencies, like other social service settings, are staffed by line workers and administrators; the training must affect both the direct skills for working with clients and procedural policies. In addition, however, these agencies include a roster of foster families, and they must be trained to work cooperatively with the child's family. It will be useful for the reader to note the similarities and differences between the training described in this situation and the training at the residential center discussed in the previous chapter, noting always that these trainers share a systemic philosophy but are working in different circumstances.

The training was conducted at three agencies, within a large urban foster care system, where administrators had expressed their interest and willingness to participate in the project.[2] The sequence, as outlined in Table 6.1, proceeded through five phases, beginning with the administrators and centered thereafter on foster care staff and foster parents, who were trained both separately and together.

Contact with Administrators

The trainers met first with agency directors and executive staff. The administrators needed more detail about the project; the trainers needed to know how the agency functioned and what the training was expected to accomplish. Practical discussions set up the specifics, including who would participate and how the training would proceed. In a general presentation to the staff at large, the trainers

[2]We wish to express our thanks to the Edna McConnell Clark Foundation and to the State of New York for grants in support of the project, and to the administrators and staffs of the cooperating agencies at the time the project was conducted.

TABLE 6.1. Training Plan and Sequence

	Foster care workers	Foster parents	Administrators
Phase I			
Contact with administrators; arrangements for training			Discussions, planning, contract
Phase II			
Staff training; four to six meetings	Framework and concepts: activities, tapes, role play, demonstration		
Phase III			
Continue staff training; begin foster parent training, three to four meetings	Work with agency cases; mapping, planning, interviews, skill building	Framework and concepts: *Training Manual for Foster Parents*	↑ Policy discussions regarding intake, visitation, case coordination, arising from case issues ↓
Phase IV			
Training of staff and foster parent teams; skill building	Combined training; work together on issues of intake, visitation, discharge, team collaboration, coordination of roles; meet as teams with agency families		
Phase V			
Training becomes in-house staff development	Foster care staff become leaders; train new staff and foster parents	Foster parents participate in training new foster parents	

described their point of view, presented the training plan, and responded to questions. Even when training is confined to a pilot group, the rest of the staff must be informed and feel included so that changes can spread later through the agency.

Selection of the social workers and foster parents who would participate was handled differently by the several agencies. One agency sought volunteers while another chose particular people; in one agency, the social workers chose foster parents who would join them, while in another the foster parents were chosen independently; and agency directors varied in the extent to which they participated in the process. This first phase inevitably looks different, from one setting to another, but it's always important to review the state of affairs with administrators as the training progresses. The trainers in our project met at intervals with administrators in order to discuss such matters as intake, visitation, and case coordination. Administrators are responsible for making policy, and if they are convinced that new procedures have value, they generally have the power to remove impediments.

Staff Training

Intensive training began with the foster care staff. The overall goal was to develop a team approach, in which the social worker and the foster parent share a viewpoint and complement each other. However, they have different roles. Foster care workers carry the professional responsibility, and the systemic approach is usually different from the way they have been working. They need to discuss the material and implement new skills within their own group first.

PHASE I

The task of these early meetings is to work on changes in attitude and framework. It's essential for the staff to broaden their ideas about who is involved in a foster care situation, to realize that the child must make a dramatic transition from one family to another, and to consider how they might encourage interaction between the two families. To establish this groundwork, our staff used experiential exercises, videotapes, didactic information, handouts, discussions, role play, and demonstration. Many of the exercises and role-play scenarios have been incorporated into a *Training Manual for Foster Parents* (P. Minuchin et al., 1990), and they are useful not only for the training of foster parents but for any professional group interested in the ecological approach (see Appendix 6.1 for Table of Contents).

As an example: An activity described in the first session of the *Manual* focuses on some details of the participant's family. Each one draws a map of his or her family, noting ages and gender, to create a simple picture of family membership and structure. Then, within small groups, they trade maps and are asked to "guess at" one developmental task for another person's family at their current stage of life (e.g., "You've got two kids in school; you probably have to keep an eye on homework and how they're doing"; or "I see you've got your father living with you and he's not so young; maybe you have to take care of him"). In the next exercise, participants imagine that the family has taken in a 5-year-old foster boy, and each one discusses the probable reaction of his or her family: What would the family expect of the child? What rules would he have to follow? How would different members of the family react if he were bossy or aggressive? Who would help him if he were scared? In other exercises, participants deal with the placement of siblings in foster care, with issues of ethnicity, visiting, and so forth.

It should be made clear to participants that the training is not oriented toward teaching them how to function as family therapists, but it's fair to point out that they are already responsible for decisions that involve an understanding of systems—how a family is functioning, what is blocking the effort to change things for the better, and so forth—and that the training is helpful for that work. Session tapes are particularly useful tools for illustrating basic ideas and sparking discussion. Since a recorded session can be stopped, backed up, and viewed again to clarify a point, it becomes possible for the trainer to illustrate the repetitive nature of family patterns and for the group to pick up what is happening (e.g., the child demands attention each time the mother and her male friend begin to argue).

Because staff workers often focus automatically on pathology, recorded sessions are also useful for demonstrating family strengths and resourcefulness. And because workers are accustomed to listening for content, it's helpful to draw attention to the nonverbal patterns that illustrate so much about family functioning: who leads the discussion, who comforts other people, who deflects an argument, and so forth. Recorded sessions should reflect the same population as the agency's clientele and contain problems typical of families with children in foster care.

PHASE II

After these basic sessions, the training focused on the skills required for connecting and empowering families: joining, searching for strength, and complementarity. Joining comes easily for trained social workers, but the search for strength and an emphasis on complementarity are more difficult. Against the background of problems that multicrisis families bring, and accustomed to the professional emphasis on pathology, workers have trouble focusing on strengths and resources. They also have difficulty with the idea of complementarity, meaning, for example, that whenever professionals are active, the clients will be passive, and that when the staff leaves space, the clients can become more active. People who are helpers by nature and profession do not find it easy to step back, leaving action and control to others.

The meeting described earlier, which brought together "Kiko," his baby brother, and their foster and biological parents, illustrates the exercise of these skills. The social worker suggested that the biological mother take over the care of the baby, and that the foster parents describe their home and family to the boys' parents. The trainer suggested that the mother share the details of her children's early development with the foster parents. The observers saw an intervention that tempered professional competence, rebalanced the usual pattern of complementarity, and empowered people who were used to being disqualified. Through simple suggestions and behavior, the trainer made space for the social worker, the social worker made space for the foster parents, and the foster parents made space for the biological parents. The tension and wariness that marked the beginning of the session dissipated over time, and, as the meeting went on, it became clear that the intake process had been flawed. If the family had been brought in for such a meeting at the start, it would have been clear that Kiko could walk and talk and knew his name, and that his regressive behavior was a reaction to separation and placement.

Foster Parent Training

Training of the foster parents began in a separate group. Foster parents have their own perspective and should be able to explore their particular task before meeting with the social workers. These first meetings should also change their sense of where they fit into the agency. In most agencies, foster parents are actively solicited and their contribution is gratefully acknowledged. Nonetheless, the definition of the job and the process of selection and instruction often convey a message of limited functions (child care) and tight control (obedience to agency rules). The child-protective motivations for monitoring and control are obvious, but training often misses a valuable opportunity: The process should empower the foster parents as important members of the service team, at the same time as it conveys basic instructions.

Almost any agency has both newly recruited and experienced foster parents. Training for the novices must not only include information about agency procedures, but also shape their view of foster care at the start, emphasizing the importance of the biological family and the breadth of their own role. New foster parents may be particularly open-minded, but if they're very critical of biological families, it's best to know that at the start.

Experienced foster parents have often taken in and released a number of children over the years, and they know the routines very well. They may either be particularly wise about parenting a foster child or especially resistant to new perspectives—and they're apt to be a little of both. If an agency is to develop a coherent approach, it's necessary to create a "refresher" experience for this group, honoring the fruits of accumulated knowledge but also expanding their understanding of the roles and attitudes the agency is now encouraging.

The *Training Manual for Foster Parents* is applicable for both new and experienced groups. It consists of a theoretical section, followed by eight training sessions (see Appendix 6.1). The sessions build a framework for understanding families, with particular emphasis on their diversity and strength and on the experience of the child and the two families when a child is placed. The activities include mapping, role play, small group work, and the discussion of vignettes concerning foster care and child development. Most foster parents have children of their own, but a review of development in the context of foster placement is a reminder that foster children of a particular age may behave differently than the family's own children. They have often had difficult experiences, and they have been uprooted.

The topic of visitation is thoroughly explored in the *Manual*. Visits between family and child are the lifeline of foster care, but foster parents may be wary of the visits. They may hold negative stereotypes or they may have heard disturbing anecdotes about intrusive parents, and they may be most comfortable with agency policies that emphasize the protection of the foster family from the child's relatives. On the other hand, we have also seen compassionate, matter-of-fact reactions from foster parents, and have heard varied suggestions for alternatives to routine visits on agency premises: for instance, a picnic in the park, a get-together at McDonald's, shared birthday parties, telephone calls, and an exchange of letters and photographs. For many foster parents, the idea of maintaining contact between families makes sense. As one foster parent remarked, "The kids handle easier if they know you like their mother."

In some respects, foster parents may be more streetwise than social workers. One exercise in the *Manual* (session 5) describes a situation in which a 7-year-old boy has been placed in foster care while his mother serves a 6-month jail term for drug charges. A group of foster parents was asked to discuss whether and how the child should be taken to visit. Social workers often have particular difficulty with this idea, but the foster parents reacted with a vigorous discussion. They agreed that the child could not be protected from knowing where his mother was, that it was important for this depressed little boy to see and talk with her, and that they would need to prepare him beforehand for the procedures and atmosphere at the prison.

Foster parents are often convinced that they have particular information unavailable to the staff, and they may be right. Myra says:

> "What's going on is . . . the agency isn't always able to see what the biological mother is doing. . . . We're the ones who have to observe. . . . Most of the time, the foster mothers have a better understanding of the families and know the parents better than the case workers, so really it's up to us."

Cara looks at the situation from a different angle. She says:

> "Some case workers look at the natural mother as a bad influence on the child, and they feel this. They're not stupid!"

Janine is less sure. She says:

> "Well, if the parent's a drug addict or something like that. . . ."

But Cara feels strongly:

> "Whether they're a drug addict, or whatever addict they are, they're still that kid's mother! They're just as human as me and

you. No matter how bad the parent is, the child wants to go back to the mother or father. You find the worst parent, the child will still want to be returned to the natural mother."

Marilyn adds:

"Well, you got some good case workers and some who are not so good. You got some who will work to the bone to unite them with the kids, and you got some who say, 'Oh, she's nothing but a crackhead . . . she's nothing but a drug user.' "

It may be useful for the workers to realize that foster parents have some unexpressed criticisms of the staff.

The Team: Training Staff and Foster Parents Together

In a sense, the preparation of these teams is the ultimate focus of the training. Social workers and foster parents will be working together with the child's family, and it's essential for them to realize that they form a system representing the agency. They will be responsible for forming a collaborative triangle that includes the birth family, and to do that successfully they should be trained together. The rationale is similar to the thinking that guides family therapists; it's understood that each individual has issues of his or her own, but the key to understanding how family members live together and deal with their problems is to work with the family as an interactive system. That reasoning guided the plan to train social workers and foster parents together, allowing them to discuss roles and develop cooperative skills in supervised sessions with the birth families.

When staff and foster parents are brought together, their task is twofold: to form cooperative teams and to work together with biological families. Teams are both powerful and complex. People who work together often complement each other's strengths, but they also face potential conflicts of turf and role. If the status of team members is different from the start, as in the case of social workers and foster parents, collaboration can be difficult. They must clarify roles and explore the boundaries of their autonomy and interdependence, even while they are forming cooperative units.

Discussions that solidify a shared perspective and prepare the team for meeting with agency families can be triggered in a variety of ways, including input from clients of the agency. Kelsey's comments, described earlier, were addressed to a combined group of social workers and foster parents in training, and they provided a detailed exposure to the frustrations and sensibilities of the birth parent. Her description led to a discussion about the impact of a foster parent's behavior on the child's relatives, the problems that arise in parenting a young child, and the ways in which a foster mother can facilitate the parent's competence. The discussion also clarified the role of the social worker, who must monitor the relationship between the two families and enter the situation if it deteriorates.

Though such discussions are important, most of the training at this phase is hands-on. Each team meets with biological families from the agency, and in each case they must create a network in which the child's family can function as a central and respected member of the triangle. In the process, they usually come to understand where they fall naturally in the division of labor, where they run into confusion, and what issues they must resolve.

It's not unusual for the team to face resentment when they first meet with family members. In the following example, the mother of three boys has become estranged from the agency in charge of her children, and the team of social worker and foster parents is attempting to reestablish contact. It's a useful example of team functioning because the social worker and foster parents were relatively experienced by that point, and the situation was well handled.

Jana had brought her children voluntarily into foster care at a point of crisis in her life. They were placed with two families on the agency's roster, and she came in regularly for visits. Because she found the setting cramped and noisy, she asked permission to take the boys outside. As a matter of policy, the request was refused. Jana was resentful, and, as the situation escalated, she broke contact and no longer came to visit.

The team decided that the foster mothers would contact Jana; they were her neighbors and the children were living in their homes. When she agreed, the team also decided that the foster parents would carry the session, though the social worker would help out if needed.

The meeting began with Jana sitting between Clara and Laura, the foster parents, while Maude, the social worker, sat slightly to the side. As everybody settled down, Jana sat with her arms folded across her chest, silent and wary. Clara spoke first. She had the oldest boy, 12-year-old Bobby, and the youngest, 5-year-old Malcolm, in her care. "Jana, I just want to tell you . . . you have two beautiful sons."

A gracious beginning. Jana smiles, nods, and relaxes a little. Laura makes a joke about James being a handful. James is 10, and has been placed separately because he's a difficult child. Jana comments that everybody petted the oldest and the youngest, but James was the middle one and had a harder time.

Clara asks now, "Do you like the way I'm taking care of your boys?" She takes it for granted that Jana has the right to judge how somebody else is caring for her children. Jana says yes, and that she knows Clara is spoiling them. It's a light comment, and they both laugh. Clara continues in a serious vein, saying that Malcolm had difficulties when he first came to live with her. "He was very emotional. I really needed to give him lots of time . . . he's stronger now."

At this point, Jana becomes an active participant. She talks about the problem of preparing the boys for leaving her. She comments that she never hid anything from Bobby, who is responsible and very smart, and that she explained the situation to the two older boys but knew that Malcolm was too young to understand. As Jana continues, it's clear that she's an intelligent, observant parent who is concerned about her children and attuned to their personalities and individual differences.

Laura joins in to talk about the difficulties she's having with James. She says, "So, I'm having a little problem with him right now. With you, when he had tantrums, the way he does . . . I mean, how did you deal with it? What did you do?"

This is a respectful vote of confidence. Laura is asking for help in solving a problem, acknowledging that Jana has experience in dealing with her son and probably has useful ideas. It's a first step toward forming a cooperative system that can pool resources on behalf of the children. Jana responds that James doesn't like people to tell him what to do, and she describes how she manages him.

By 15 minutes into their meeting, the three parents were discussing the children and the realities of the situation. Although the behavior of the foster parents was spontaneous, it was based on their understanding that this contact was important, and it reflected the skills they had developed for conveying respect and interest. As a result, they tapped the strength and knowledge of the mother in a very short time and began the process of constructive communication.

The social worker was present but silent through most of the meeting. If the foster parents had been less skillful or Jana less responsive, she would necessarily have been more active. Since that was not the case, her role was to facilitate by holding back. As events unfold in the future, however, she will be responsible for evaluating progress and carrying the case forward.

Situations of this kind have brought policy questions to the fore. Could procedures be evaluated on a case-by-case basis? Were there creative ways to establish sequences in the procedures so that, for instance, parents like Jana might move from visits at the agency to outside excursions, accompanied first by a foster parent and then without supervision? Matters brought up with administrators were sometimes facilitated and sometimes not, but learning at the staff level was evident. The team work of social workers and foster parents, as they met with birth families, became more consistently effective, and in some settings, participants in the program went on to train others at their agency in this way of working.

Finishing and Moving On

During the several years of the project, the trainers had dealt with personnel at all levels of the agencies, but the project was focused primarily on helping the staff to think and work differently so the biological families would become more functional and reunification more probable. Staff training with that focus is always essential. However, training in itself does not solve the organizational issues of foster care. Over the recent decade or so, concern for the child's experience has moved more firmly into the spotlight, and it has become ever more evident that flaws in the larger system impede the journey toward an optimal outcome. The second project, presented below, centers on these factors, and on work that is addressed to bringing about constructive change.

A FAMILY-FOCUSED APPROACH TO PERMANENCY

Legislation at the federal level specifies goals and guidelines for social programs. In the area of foster care, the Adoption and Safe Families Act (ASFA), passed by Congress in 1997, set a stringent time frame for the resolution of foster care cases. Based on a consideration of the realities of "child time," it stipulated that if a child has been in foster care for 15 out of the last 22 months, agencies must institute procedures for terminating parental rights and moving toward adoption. At about the same time, policies shifted at the local level in New York City, where the Administration for Children's Services (ACS) articulated a "family-to-family" philosophy of service in relation to foster care.

The Foster Care Project, directed by Colapinto and summarized briefly in the opening pages of this chapter, was clearly consistent with these policies, since it combined a family focus with a concern for permanency. A consultation contract with ACS allowed Colapinto and his associates to participate in the foster care network, observing the details of the process and working to implement a family-focused approach to permanency.[3]

Presentation of this work is separated into three areas: connections and empowerment; child time as a developmental issue; and the system network.

Connections and Empowerment

Any program with an ecological point of view necessarily emphasizes connections. In the foster care situation, connections among various parts of the system and empowerment of the biological family are parts of the basic philosophy, and this project continued the earlier work of strengthening those aspects. There were new formulations and emphases, however, regarding the contact between families, the relational aspects of service planning, and the connection between child and birth parents during the period of placement.

Contact between Families

Procedures for facilitating contact between the families were described in connection with the first project. In the second project, a

[3]The Foster Care Project was housed at the Ackerman Institute for the Family and initially funded through grants from the Rauch Foundation and the Child Welfare Fund. In 2000, a multiyear contract provided for training, curriculum development, and technical assistance to the Administration for Children's Services and its contract agencies. In addition to Jorge Colapinto, as Director, project associates included, at various times, Neelam Al-Angurli, Nancy Douzinas, Richard Johnson, Kathy Lecube, Catherine Lewis, Mary Ann Quinson, and Gloria Zuss.

new feature was added: a focus on the tension, suspicion, and antagonism that is typical in the relations between families, and a direct approach to working with that reality.

Mutual distrust between birth and foster families is the natural expression of an unnatural arrangement. Both families must deal with uncertainty and paradoxical conditions. The foster parents are asked to give unconditional love to the child but not to become too attached because the child is supposed to return to his or her own family, though they should keep open the possibility of adoption at a later point. The birth parents are expected to give up the child and prepare themselves to function as better parents in the future, though they will have restricted contact with the child while they are doing so and may not, in the end, have custody.

This odd situation calls for "straight talk"—the acknowledgment of differences in the perspectives of the two families, and of the distrust that is almost inevitable in their perceptions of each other. The point should be made, in a variety of ways, that connection does not necessarily mean harmony. It's not necessary for families to like each other; the more relevant and viable task is to talk to each other. Rather than keeping the families apart and anesthetizing their contacts, workers need to concentrate on channeling emotional intensity in the service of useful communication.

Consider the following incident:

Ms. Sanchez, a foster mother, calls the agency supervisor at the last minute to say that she cannot bring 5-year-old Leo for a visit with his father.

SUPERVISOR: Would it be OK for the father to call you when he comes to the agency?

MS. SANCHEZ: No! He's going to yell at me.

SUPERVISOR: What would you do if he yells at you?

MS. SANCHEZ: He's done that before. I will probably yell back, and hang up.

SUPERVISOR: And if he talks nice?

MS. SANCHEZ: He won't. I know. But if he's nice I would explain to him what happened. Maybe reschedule.

SUPERVISOR: So he has a choice, doesn't he? Remember when we talked about choices, and how important it is that the two of you have a line of communication?

MS. SANCHEZ: Yeah . . . OK, tell him to call me.

When Mr. Romero, the father, arrives at the agency and is told that the visit has been cancelled, he confronts the supervisor.

MR. ROMERO: The woman did it again!

SUPERVISOR: I know. I talked to Ms. Sanchez and told her you might call.

MR. ROMERO: No. I won't talk to her. It's your job. You tell her she's supposed to bring my child here.

SUPERVISOR: Sure, I can do that. But Ms. Sanchez knows that already, and remember that we talked about how important it is that you talk to each other, most of all when something needs to be cleared up. Of course you're upset. I would be upset if I were you, but what do you think is better for Leo? That you don't call Ms. Sanchez, and next time there will be a lot of tension between the two of you?

MR. ROMERO: It's not going to do any good. I'm too upset to talk to her.

SUPERVISOR: Sure. I would be upset if I were you. Don't you think she should know that? If you don't call her, she may think you don't care.

After further discussion, Mr. Romero decides that he will call Ms. Sanchez. The supervisor reminds Mr. Romero, as he has done on similar occasions, that he has a choice. "You can just vent your anger on the phone, or you can let Ms. Sanchez know that you're disappointed and you expect to see your child some other day this week." Mr. Romero chooses the second alternative, and after finishing the phone conversation, says to the supervisor, "She's OK."

The supervisor has resisted the demand to buffer the situation by taking over, and has led the two parents to a communication that is more satisfying for the adults and better for the child.

Relational Focus in Service Planning

When a child is taken into custody, the courts set goals for changes that must occur before the family can be reunited. Typically, child and parent are set going along parallel tracks: the child to adapt to a new home, the parent to attend mandated services. It is assumed that events will proceed sequentially. After the parent has completed the services, presumably becoming a better parent without further experience in parenting, the family can be reunited. Until then, parents and children are expected to remain attached in some virtual way. But isolation begets something different. The ties that bind parent and child dissolve, and they become attached to their immediate and separate realities. The arrangement of parallel tracks has actually resulted in patterns that disconnect (Colapinto, 1995).

To set up a different planning process, a new form, labeled "Reunification Plan," was drawn up. The form focuses on the maintenance and development of the parents' connection to the child. The entries describe parental strengths and an assessment of the problems or conditions to be corrected, as well as goals, target dates, tasks to be undertaken, and services needed. An example for one family appears in Figure 6.2.

The form is intended to shape the way workers think about their clients from the beginning of their contact, using relational terminology to emphasize connections. Parents' "availability to the child" points to the quality of their relationship, as does the "emotional connection" to the child, the "support" from extended family or community, and such negatives as abuse or neglect, which are neither static matters nor resident only in the parent, but are issues of the relationship between parent and child. The fact that each item must be considered in terms of goals and tasks for maintenance and development makes the process of assessment more detailed, enhancing the likelihood that services will be selected thoughtfully rather than automatically.

Contact between Parent(s) and Child during Placement

Keeping child and parent connected through the placement is a continuing challenge. It requires recognition that the relationship is a psychological need, rather than a problem that must be calmed and diverted, and that the parent's attachment to the child is an asset rather than a nuisance. There are countless examples of situations where parent–child visits are inconvenient or difficult to arrange; without an understanding of their importance, they are postponed or cut short. The court has ordered, for instance, that Kayla's visits with her daughter should occur "as frequently as possible, but should be closely supervised." Kayla works and can only visit on Saturdays, but the agency has staffing problems on the weekend so visits are scheduled twice a month instead of weekly. Regrettably, nobody considers this a problem.

Agencies often regard visits as just an opportunity for family members to "see" each other, rather than a vital part of sustaining their relationship and improving interaction. The message is not lost on the parents themselves. Donna has been offered a second weekly visit with her children. During the visits, she often spent time chatting with the workers rather than focusing on the children, and, after a time, she began to miss visits, saying she has a lot to do and will have time for the children when they return to her. In Melanie's case, an acceptable place for the family to live is the required condition for the return of her son. The housing agency has moved her up on the waiting list, but when an apartment became available Melanie turned it down because it was a long ride to the school she planned to attend. The court extends foster care so the search can continue. Nobody has alerted Melanie to the risks of postponing reunification, or helped her to weigh the relative advantages of earlier reunification against a more desirable apartment.

When parents like Donna and Melanie drift away from their children, it's customary to blame their lack of concern. However, a wider lens often reveals the pull of competing interests: the search for housing or a job, a new boyfriend, even drugs. Simply waiting for the parent to demonstrate motivation, or the lack of it, will not do; workers need to be proactive, reinforcing the parent–child connection so it can withstand the centrifugal pull of other forces.

The creation of a new form, labeled "Progress Note: Observed Visit," has set up a guideline for recording the details of a visit between parents and child (see Figure 6.3 for an example of one case). This form records who is present at the visit, the goals, the relationship between parent(s) and child during the visit, and the ways in which the parent(s) interact with the child while they are together. It also provides for a summary concerning improvement in the parent–child relationship, and indicates whether the observation has been discussed with the parent(s).

Clearly, the usefulness of such a form goes beyond the value of keeping a record for each family. It changes the way a worker thinks about a visit and observes what is happening. It focuses the worker's attention, highlights the importance of small interactions between

(text continues on p. 168)

Reunification Plan		Parent's name: *Malena García*			Date: *Jan. 10*
(A) PARENTAL STRENGTHS TO BE MAINTAINED OR DEVELOPED					
1. Strength	**2. Current level** of parental strength	**3. Goals:** Observable indicators of maintenance/development of strength	**4. Target dates**	**5. Tasks** to be undertaken by parents, foster parents, and others, to help maintain/develop strengths	**6. Services** needed to develop strengths
Available to child?	*Has not visited since child was placed 3 months ago*	*2-hour visits twice a week and daily phone calls*	*Immediately*	*Mother will visit as indicated. Foster mother will participate in visits.*	*Structured visits, including coaching and debriefing*
Emotionally connected with child?	*Unknown due to lack of observed contact*	*Noticing/responding to child's cues*	*April*	*Interact with child during visits.*	*" " " "*
Able to meet child's material, educational, psychosocial, medical needs?	*(+) Meets material & educational needs* *(−) Allows for excessive physical punishment* *(−) Minimizes medical needs*	*Supporting adjustment of child to foster home*	*Immediately*	*"Passing of the baton": Mother and foster mother will talk jointly to child.*	
		Guiding in nonviolent ways	*April*	*Interact with child during visits.*	
		Participating actively in medical treatment of child	*Immediately*	*Mother will attend medical appointments; caseworker will obtain necessary permissions from medical personnel.*	
Utilizes prescribed services?	*Attends parenting skills course, not domestic violence counseling program*	*Attending all prescribed services*	*February*	*Since original referral to domestic violence program does not meet mother's needs, agency will address relevant issues (see below, "Unsafe environment") in its own parenting skills program.*	*Expanded parenting skills program*
Has extended family and/or community supportive of parent?	*Supported by sister, isolated from rest of family*	*Expand network of support*	*April*	*Sister will mediate between parent and rest of family. Agency will include negotiating family conflict in parenting skills program.*	*Expanded parenting skills program*

(B) PARENT'S BEHAVIORS/CONDITIONS TO BE CORRECTED					
1. Behaviors/ conditions	**2. Describe** specific behaviors or conditions	**3. Goals:** Observable indicators of corrected behavior/ condition	**4. Target date**	**5. Tasks** to be undertaken by parents, foster parents, and others, to help correct behaviors/conditions	**6. Services** needed to correct conditions
Neglect or abuse?	Allowed her boyfriend to discipline her child which led to the child's arm being fractured	Watchful vigilance of the child's safety. Self-sufficiency in disciplining the child.	April	Mother will become more acquainted with and committed to her son's needs for structure and will learn to discipline without resorting to violent ways or "helpers."	Increased visitation (at least twice a week), in a setting where mother can practice parenting. Parenting skills program
Alcohol or drug abuse?	N/A				
Other physical and/or mental health problems?	N/A				
Unsafe physical environment?	Because of child's placement and breakup with boyfriend, mother is at risk of becoming homeless	Stable housing	April	Mother, extended family, and agency will work together to secure housing.	
Unsafe psychosocial environment?	Mother's boyfriend was violent to the child. Has since left the home	Continuing violence-free environment for the child.	April	Mother's sister, other family members will help her reconcile need for violence-free home for her son with need for adult companionship. Agency will add this issue to parenting skills program. Agency and extended family will work together on helping mother gain financial independence so she can be freer in choosing male companions.	Expanded parenting skills program

FIGURE 6.2. Example of a completed Reunification Plan.

165

Progress Note: OBSERVED VISIT

Level of observation:	Location of visit: *Agency*
☐ Strict supervision ☒ Monitoring	Observed by: *L.M.*

Scheduled: from *2* to *3:30* | **Actual time:** from *2* to *3:30*

Scheduled participants:	Relationship to child:	On time/late/not present:	Explanations/ comments:
Malena García	*Birth mother*		*Everybody was on time.*
Estela López	*Foster mother*		
Luis García	*Foster child*		
Sara García	*Maternal aunt*		

PRE-VISIT

☒ Parent(s) had specific goals that they wanted to accomplish in visit.
☒ Foster parent and/or worker alerted the birth parent(s) to specific needs of the child(ren) for this visit.
☐ Other interactions prior to the visit influencing the visit positively or negatively.

Describe: *Birth mother wants to refamiliarize herself with the son. This is the second visit since the mother started visits, which was three months after the child was placed. Both the foster parent and the worker have alerted the parents to the anxiety that Luis has manifested about the visit.*

Initial responses of child(ren) and parent(s) to each other (*Calm, Happy, Sad, Sullen, Indifferent, Anxious, etc.*):

Describe: *Luis was happy to see his mother and aunt, but also anxious. The aunt was more demonstrative than the mother in greeting Luis.*

DURING THE VISIT

Child(ren)'s overall relationship to parent(s) (*Comfortable, Eager, Apathetic, Overexcited, Avoiding, Resistant, etc.*):

Describe: *Luis was initially excited and wanting to attract the attention of his mother and aunt. As the grownups started to interact more among themselves, Luis sat in the middle of the room playing by himself.*

(continued)

FIGURE 6.3. Example of a completed Progress Note: Observed Visit.

Parent(s)' interaction with child(ren):	Check:	Give examples of parent(s) actions, and/or help offered to them.
1. Were responsive to the child(ren)	☐ Yes, spontaneously ☒ Yes, with help ☐ No	*Mother tended to lay back and interact with the grownups in the room more than with Luis. However she responded well to the caseworker's efforts to redirect her attention to Luis.*
2. Provided structure and/ or guidance	☐ Yes, spontaneously ☐ Yes, with help ☒ No ☐ Not needed	*The foster mother, and sometimes the aunt, provided structure and guidance for Luis throughout the visit.*
3. Initiated age-relevant activities	☐ Yes, spontaneously ☐ Yes, with help ☒ No	*None of the adults took the initiative in this respect.*
4. Dealt effectively with the child(ren)'s problem behaviors	☒ Yes, spontaneously ☐ Yes, with help ☐ No ☐ Not needed	*At one point when Luis was making too much noise with a toy truck, his mother said that if he could not play quietly he would have to put the track back in the box, and Luis quieted down.*
5. Encouraged interaction among the siblings	☐ Yes, spontaneously ☐ Yes, with help ☐ No ☒ Not applicable	
6. Helped the child(ren) separate at the end of the visit	☐ Yes, spontaneously ☒ Yes, with help ☐ No ☐ Not needed	*10 minutes before the scheduled end for the visit, the aunt started talking to Luis about the next visit, but then the mother took over, helped Luis with their coats, and walked him to the outside.*

Other observations on parent–child interaction:
The adults interacted more with each other than with the child.

SUMMARY ASSESSMENT. Compared to previous visit, the quality of parent–child relationship has

☒ Improved   ☐ Deteriorated   ☐ Not changed

Describe: *Mother provided effective guidance when Luis's play became too noisy. In future sessions she must be helped to take more initiative and be more responsible to Luis.*

At the end of the visit:

☒ Observations were discussed with parent(s).

☐ Observations were not discussed with parent(s).

Describe: *Caseworker shared the observations about the improvements and what still needs to be done. The mother was in agreement but said she was still unsure about what was expected from her in the visits.*

parent and child, and encourages the thoughtful evaluation of what has changed and what must still be worked on.

Child Time as a Developmental Concern

Even with a shift in attitudes and procedures, a successful reunification of the biological family is not a certainty. This project, therefore, has focused on developing a process that prepares from the beginning for alternative outcomes.

It has always been clear that foster placement is about the care and protection of children, yet the child's perspective has not been at the center of the planning or the pace, and the workings of the system have created a culture of impermanence that jeopardizes child growth. Healthy growth depends, basically, on the relationship to caregivers, the stability of the world around the child, and the response of people to the child's changing needs and capacities. Most of us understand that "attachment" implies a sense of emotional security, and that it stems from the way in which adults care for and comfort the child. What may be less familiar is the associated idea that the child's sense of a predictable world begins with this relationship; with the experience that things happen as expected, and that signals of distress will bring people who feed, soothe, and relieve discomfort. Realistically, that expectation must be modified somewhat, as the child grows older, but the basic sense that events are predictable and adults will respond helpfully to one's changing needs is the anchor of emotional security.

Children in foster care have often come from situations that don't fit these conditions very well, and the foster care process, by its very nature, creates further disruptions. With separation and placement, previous attachments are interrupted and the environment becomes unpredictable. Beyond what is inevitable, however, the workings of the system tend to compound the problem. Children experience delays, promises that aren't kept, recurrent separations and reunions, and expectations that multiple loyalties will somehow be sustained through it all. The process moves according to adult time: the length of the drug program; the time it takes to get on the court docket; the search for appropriate housing; the paperwork; the overcrowded schedule of the workers; and the expectation that the placement can always be extended if there is uncertainty about the appropriate action. Meanwhile, the child is in limbo, lingering in a situation of impermanence. Some children move about within the system indefinitely until they are old enough to graduate out, having formed no permanent ties either with their original families or through adoption into a new family.

In a family-focused approach to permanency, as represented by this project, the value of "child time" is upheld every step of the way. Agency staff are reminded that their mission is to bring foster care to a safe and timely conclusion, and that it is not in the interest of the child to follow the tradition of sequential planning, in which alternative outcomes are considered only after a decision has been made that the original goal cannot be met.

When workers and families meet for the first time to assess the situation and develop a service plan, the point is made that it isn't good for the child to live in an unpredictable world, and that it's important to look ahead toward a permanent resolution. Within a relatively short time, months rather than years, agencies and families must arrive at a permanency plan. The strong preference in almost any case is to return the child to the family, and all parties will be working constantly toward that end. However, since reunification is not an absolute certainty, they must also consider back-up possibilities, such as adoption, custody, or guardianship. It's necessary to talk openly about the alternatives, even while reunification efforts are proceeding, rather than denying reality and tabling discussion until a crisis arises. With the needs of the child at the forefront, possible outcomes are clarified at the start, time boundaries are firmly indicated, and the stage is set for concurrent rather than sequential planning.

It's important to emphasize that this approach does not favor child needs over those of the family. That is a false dichotomy, with advocates arguing for one position or the other and making it difficult to break the impasse that leads to chronic foster care. What is necessary is to keep the child at the center of the situation while providing the parents with information about the time frame, possible outcomes, and choices, even while the issues that have brought about placement are being attended to. Most families want to parent their own children; direct information that helps them understand the reality of their situation and the consequences of possible choices is a respectful and productive way to support the family as a system.

As time goes on, both the foster and birth families need to know where they are in the process and how things are moving. In the training and guidelines set up by this project, both families are involved in designing relevant service plans and are reminded at intervals through reviews and feedback that the clock is ticking, both legally and developmentally. Birth parents are helped to consider the implications of their choices (e.g., not accepting the apartment that's offered will delay your child's return home) and to understand the specific obstacles to reunification (e.g., skipping visits creates the impression that you're not interested). Both families are reminded that some parenting functions can take place even if parents and child are not living together (e.g., meeting the child's teacher, attending medical appointments, discussing important issues with the child). If all goes well, the visiting plan is monitored so that it's appropriately progressive, moving from supervised visits at the agency to other places, times, and conditions.

Whatever the final resolution, the intention is to provide the child with continuity, and with the sense of a network that is supportive and dependable. Children should not have to lose people they are attached to as the by-product of attaining a permanent home. Facilitating contact between families during the period of placement eases the period of transition, when a permanent decision is made, and increases the likelihood that connections will continue in the future.

The System Network

The Multiple Sources of Blockage

It must be clear, at this point, that the blockage of productive movement occurs at many levels. Some problems arise at the agency level, where arrangements are handled and the practical issues of staffing, scheduling, and funding may interfere with primary goals. Like Kayla, whose visits with her daughter were limited for reasons of space and supervision, Jason's mother could see her son only biweekly because of crowded conditions at the agency. In this case, however, other options had been considered but were turned down by the families. The foster family was not willing to have mother and son meet at their home, and Jason's mother would not allow placement with his paternal grandmother because she and her mother-in-law did not get along. Blockage came originally from conditions at the agency but was compounded by the two families. All had reacted in terms of their own issues rather than a concern for the child's connection to his mother.

In other cases, a family perspective is blocked by networks

within the larger system: medical, educational, protective, and/or legal services assembled in relation to different aspects of the situation. Often a professional staff has never been alerted to the meaning of connections within a family or the importance of time from the child's perspective. Sometimes they are simply following traditional procedures. Lawyers, for instance generally prefer that the two families not communicate because of a potential "conflict of interest." If abuse is alleged, the child's lawyer may object to reunification efforts until the parents admit their culpability—something the parents' lawyer may be urging them not to do.

For their part, teachers don't think to communicate with two sets of parents, nor do medical personnel, who tend to focus on treatment of the sick child. It happens only if someone raises the suggestion and offers a rationale. Even judges may contribute to the confusion. Frustrated by the real or perceived inefficiency of the agencies, they may become de-facto planners, though they are not necessarily wiser or more effective. When Wanda's infant was born with an addiction to cocaine, for instance, the judge ordered Wanda into a program that forbids contact with the baby for at least a month and postpones the possibility of reunification until the end of the 18-month program. When the agency worker requested an exception from the guidelines, explaining that "it's a way of protecting the bond of mother and baby," the judge replied, "The baby will have time to bond with the mother once she's sober." Given the hierarchy of power in the system, workers learn to shortcut the process, noting that it's a waste of time to seek a different outcome since the judge is not likely to change a ruling.

Interventions

It would be desirable, of course, to approach change at all these levels simultaneously, but the system is too complex and too static. It's more realistic to intervene at any level that becomes accessible, offering concrete recommendations and challenging constraints imposed from elsewhere that interfere with changes acceptable to the staff.

The process of planning services offers a useful example. The process is meant to match services to needs after a careful assessment, but, in practice, the needs evaluation is often skipped over, replaced by an automatic pairing of the "reason for placement" (drug abuse, domestic violence, inadequate housing) with the well-known roster of available services (drug treatment, anger management, housing assistance, and a course in parenting skills for good measure). Insiders refer to this as the "cookie cutter approach." The revision of guidelines for assessment and service planning, as described earlier in the chapter, has created a more detailed and personal process, moving workers and families toward a plan that is more relevant to the particular case. Sometimes that involves a search outside the usual pathways, as in the following situation:

Nineteen-year-old Marie is living with her 2-year old son, Andy, and her mother, Yvette, in Yvette's home. Though they usually get along, there are stormy periods, and after one confrontation in which a knife is brandished, Andy is removed from his grandmother's home and placed in foster care. Marie moves out of the house and goes to live with friends nearby. A few days later, when things have calmed down, both Marie and Yvette request that Andy be taken out of the foster home and placed in Yvette's custody. The workers hesitate and then call a meeting of the two women, the agency worker, and a consultant from the project to develop a service plan. The core of the discussion is as follows:

CONSULTANT: What do you need to do to get Andy back?

YVETTE: We need to go to anger management.

CONSULTANT: Together?

YVETTE: (*after visually checking with the worker*) No, separate groups.

CONSULTANT: Who else are you angry at, other than Marie?

YVETTE: Nobody. I'm not angry at her either.

CONSULTANT: Marie, who else are you angry at?

MARIE: Just my mother.

CONSULTANT: (*to worker*) I think they should go to anger management together. They don't have any other anger to manage.

WORKER: But that's not how it works. The anger management program won't take both of them together.

Here the consultant has used the assessment process to slow things down, make a relational point, and move the worker toward a plan that challenges the way things are usually done. In this case, the worker went looking for and found a program willing to work with the two women together—a resolution that held promise for a better and speedier outcome for Andy as well as his relatives.

Of course, the effort by workers to change the usual procedures may well prove frustrating. The social worker who appealed to the judge on behalf of Wanda and her baby was met by a flat refusal. In a sense, however, the fact that the agency asked the judge to review his decision introduced a challenge into the system, interrupting the automatic nature of such mandates and suggesting there were other rational possibilities. Experienced social work supervisors often anticipate a decision and accept it in advance: "I would recommend that Jessica go back with her mom," said one supervisor, "but this judge is antiparent and she won't go for that. Period." The supervisor's recommendation is understandable to save time and disappointment, but as a result of that "period," judges who don't think in terms of family attachments never hear about them. The worker's request to send Wanda to an outpatient program may, in fact, have replaced the period with a semicolon; some months later, the same judge referred a family to a rehab program for mother and child.

Two Illustrative Cases

Interventions that challenge accepted practices, and that involve many people at different levels of the system, are hard work, but the effort is necessary and sometimes effective. The following cases describe the effort to bring about constructive change by working step by step with the different parties who render service and make decisions.

The Case of Charna

A meeting has been called at a private foster care agency to discuss the case of 1-year-old Charna, who was placed in foster care at birth because she and her mother were HIV positive. The discussion group is to consider the service plan, which is scheduled for review every 6 months. Are child and family receiving the necessary services? Are the parents cooperative? What else must be done before the child can be discharged from foster care? The consultant knows there is some tendency to "spin wheels" at such meetings, to review details from the beginning and continue current efforts whether they are working or not. He sees his role as helping participants to look carefully at the current situation, to consider new ideas, if necessary, and to move along toward the goal.

It is a mixed group. Agency personnel include the caseworker, the supervisor, and the nurse, as well as a parent advocate—usually a former client who has successfully regained custody of her children. The latter is expected to understand the perspective of the birth parent and may either support or challenge the caseworker. Also present are Charna's mother, Dana, the case manager from the city's child welfare agency, the consultant, and a meeting facilitator—a "third-party reviewer" who has no involvement in the case and will presumably provide an objective point of view. The advantages and disadvantages of this mix are well known: multiple perspectives that enrich the situation are combined with unspoken hierarchies and issues of turf.

As the meeting starts, the facilitator asks the caseworker for her report. She reviews the services briefly, and then focuses on the one aspect of the plan that has not been completed: the mother has not been attending a course for learning how to deal with her HIV condition. An argument ensues. Dana says the worker had referred her to programs located in unsafe neighborhoods and that, on her own, she has found and attended a support group for mothers with HIV. The worker maintains that a support group does not provide the expert medical information that the mother needs, and she dismisses the issue of safety as an excuse.

The facilitator breaks the tension by asking the nurse for her input. The latter reports on the work she has been doing with the mother and daughter. She says that Dana participates wholeheartedly in activities designed to help her understand the medical needs of her daughter, and that she seems to be taking good care of her own medical condition. When the nurse finishes, the facilitator moves to a different issue: planning for the next 6 months, starting with the question of whether the goal of reunification should be maintained. All agree that the baby will eventually be going back to her mother.

At this point, the consultant reminds the participants that the purpose of the review is to figure out what else needs to happen so that the child can be discharged from foster care. It is actually the function of case managers from the child welfare agency to call attention to the permanency needs of the child, but in many cases, as here, they take a more limited role, monitoring the provision of prescribed services and overseeing the safety of the child in the foster home. The consultant enters to model a more goal-directed approach. He points out a contradiction: People agree the baby will return to the mother, but they have not resolved the question of whether that's contingent on the mother's attendance at an educational medical program. Since the time frame will soon expire, they must reach one of three conclusions: (1) that the mother needs to comply with the requirement; (2) that the requirement will be dropped from the service plan; or (3) that an alternative permanency plan for the baby must be developed. The consultant is pushing the group to confront the conflicts they're avoiding, noting that this evasion is at the expense of child time, which requires decisions and resolutions.

The caseworker and mother begin to argue again, and the parent advocate enters to challenge the worker: "Why don't you tell it like it is? You think she's in denial, and that's why she needs that program!" The worker replies, "It's not what I think. It's what the service plan says." The discussion that follows is a reminder of how information gets lost or distorted; how mandates survive longer than their rationale; and how staff turnover compounds the problem. The requirement that Dana must attend an HIV program came from the intake interview. Dana told the worker that she had not revealed her HIV status to her family, a fact considered evidence of denial. In the system's automatic association of particular problems with particular services (the cookie-cutter approach), "denial" required "HIV education." Though Dana had subsequently talked with her family and been an active participant in learning about the medical needs of her daughter and herself, the recorded requirement had a life of its own and did not change. The current worker had not been present at intake, had access only to the record, and knew nothing of the original rationale.

The review process in itself does not guarantee thoughtful evaluation, but if it is characterized by a sense of urgency on behalf of child and family, it can generate creative ideas and a progressive plan. In this case, participants at the meeting responded to the formulation of clear and necessary choices. They discussed their options, agreed that the requirement should be dropped from the service plan, and outlined the steps for reuniting Charna with her mother within the next 3 months.

The Case of Roby

The case of Roby illustrates the blockage created by power hierarchies and multiple perspectives within the system, as well as the ways
in which communication, persistence, and compromise can resolve
differences. Again, the effort is on behalf of the child, whose developmental clock continues to tick while professionals and parents are in
a stalemate.

Roby has been in foster care since he was 5 months old, when he
was diagnosed with shaken baby syndrome. His parents deny
responsibility for the injuries but have not been able to provide a satisfactory alternate explanation. After 6 months of placement, the
case is still legally in the fact-finding stage, meaning that the court
has not yet determined whether the parents have abused the child.

According to the initial service plan, visits must take place at the
agency and be supervised by the caseworker until the judge autho-
rizes otherwise, and the parents must receive training in parental
skills. The latter is a generic recommendation applied to the gamut of
cases from mild neglect to severe abuse. In the view of the consultant,
it illustrates the absence of "straight talk," in this case, and is apt to
block the road to permanency at a later point. If parents are suspected of abuse, they should be helped either to admit responsibility
or to collaborate in finding a different explanation. Otherwise, they
may comply dutifully with the mandate only to find later that it is
not considered sufficient.

In the 6-month review, the foster care agency considers that
there has been enough progress in their work with the parents to
request the judge's permission for unsupervised visits. The case manager from the city agency objects, noting that the law guardian for
the child has said there can be no move toward reunification until the
parents admit responsibility for the baby's injuries. From a clinical
point of view, the judgment of the agency should prevail. The caseworker holds a master's degree in social work; has worked with the
parents as a couple, individually, and as a threesome with their baby;
and has produced full reports on the progress of the case. The law
guardian has no training in social work, has never met the parents,
and has seen the baby only sporadically. It's evident, however, that
the opinion of the law guardian will carry more weight with the
judge in his or her ruling on unsupervised visits.

The consultant knows that there is a power differential between
lawyers and social workers, and that the law guardian will not attend

a review session or discuss the merits of her position with everybody else. Aside from time constraints, attorneys tend to keep their distance from people on the other side. The consultant goes to the law guardian's office, therefore, to talk over the current situation and ask her some questions. What does the law guardian need to see happening before she will agree to unsupervised visits? She first says the admission of responsibility by the parents is essential, because "as long as they deny they have a problem, the baby will not be safe with them." On second thought, however, she accepts the idea that there are many possible reasons why parents may refuse to take responsibility, including the fear of legal consequences. "If I were their lawyer," she concedes, "I would advise them against admitting."

The consultant asks the law guardian if there's something the parents can do, short of admitting responsibility, that would alleviate her concerns. She comments that what is really bothering her is that the agency is "pro-parents," and that the caseworker may be naively taken in by the family. She would be more comfortable if the parents were seen by a therapist outside the agency.

With the permission of the law guardian, the consultant informs the caseworker and supervisor, who are understandably dismayed. They believe that their work has been going well, that it's best to coordinate all the services for a family under one roof, and that a referral for therapy outside the agency would be demoralizing for the parents as well as themselves. But they also understand that the alternative is a protracted power struggle with the law guardian, adding months to the child's stay in foster care and causing additional strain on the family. The options are discussed with the parents, and their responses are immediate. "I'll do whatever it takes to get my child back," says the father, and the mother comes up with a clever question: "Shouldn't we go to see somebody that the law guardian trusts?" Consulted by phone, the law guardian says she simply wants somebody from outside the agency who can form a fresh and objective impression of the parents.

From that point, matters proceed apace. The parents are referred to a psychotherapist at a community mental health agency, and the law guardian agrees to write a letter detailing the areas she would like covered in the report. The rest of the group meets with the therapist to discuss the reasons for the referral and the concerns of the law guardian. Six weeks later, in a court hearing, the law guardian supports the initiation of unsupervised visits and permission is legally granted.

These examples describe moments in time, taken out of the longer process of placement, review, and permanency decisions. They illustrate the details that go into moving things along, when the process is blocked by arguments and postponements that frustrate the adults and victimize the child. It has been the job of the consultants to challenge nonproductive habits and encourage straight talk, acting in the role of stimulator and go-between to keep the reality of child time and the goal of permanent resolution in the forefront. Eventually, such a role must be taken over by personnel within the system, whose job will be to encourage the integration of such attitudes and procedures into all aspects of the foster care enterprise.

WHAT ENABLES A NEW APPROACH TO SURVIVE?

Despite the uphill struggle, our model has had a lasting impact on foster care practices in a variety of settings, and we can raise the question, again, of what factors help to sustain a family perspective over time. Two new factors were suggested by the foster care projects:

- Emphasis on connecting elements of the system.
- The creation of concrete tools and procedures for staff use.

Four factors discussed in the earlier chapter appeared relevant in the foster care situation as well:

- The support of social policies.
- Adaptability.
- Leadership commitment.
- Intensive family-oriented training and supervision.

Emphasis on Connecting Elements of the System

One of the most disturbing aspects of service delivery, as it is generally organized, is that the different elements travel along parallel tracks. Though staff members in the different areas are working with the same clients, there's little recognition that they are part of an interrelated system. Each group assesses what is needed, creates a plan of services, and interacts with clients within the limited boundaries of their own domain. By highlighting an ecological model for foster care, our work has challenged this structure, and through emphasizing the systemic features of the training, we have learned that connections among disparate elements promote a systems approach that can endure.

The foster care model described in this chapter invokes the concept of a cooperative triangle with three groupings: the overall system, which brings all three parts together; the subsystem of social worker and foster family, which must work cooperatively to make the birth family part of the triangle; and the members of the two families, who must find a way to relate and communicate on behalf of the child.

The important point of the model, in practical terms, is that the training program established these connections de facto. Social workers and foster parents were trained in a combined group, developing hands-on experience as a team. The two sets of parents were brought together to share information and work on problem solving. Members of the triangle met together to establish a cooperative network. By working within these several structures, proponents of the model were connecting different parts of the system and communicating the message that the elements are more effective when they function in combination with each other.

Of course, the relevant connections go beyond the central participants, involving workers from different organizations who serve different functions in relation to the same case. If they have never collaborated, they may have little understanding of how their requirements and practices affect the clients. The staff of a drug treatment program, for instance, is likely to have a different perspective than the staff of a foster care agency, and neither group of workers may understand that their competing demands confuse the client. A meeting between representatives from both organizations is often marked by tension, but it is potentially more productive than contacting the two groups separately in order to explain the situation and broker a solution. A combined meeting illustrates by its very structure that all are concerned with the same client, and it is apt to have positive repercussions beyond the particular case.

As described in the previous chapter, the consultant working with the perinatal project created multidisciplinary meetings to discuss the issues that were important for a particular client and her family. And, during the second project described in this chapter, the consultants moved about the system bringing people together who had generally followed procedures that were unilateral and sequential. The possibility that a systemic approach will endure is enhanced if the intervention activates connections among the component parts and teaches the staff that such connections are essential.

The Creation of Concrete Tools and Procedures for Staff Use

The work of service personnel is organized, and sometimes dominated, by forms to be filled out and procedures to be followed. These tools are meant to ensure that the process is thorough and helpful. In practice, however, they often become part of the problem rather than the path to desirable solutions. Any form carries a message. If data concerning pathology and problems are required to fill the page, that is the mindset conveyed to the workers; if the workers are asked to gather information about family composition and strengths, the message is different.

Our teams enter a situation with a philosophy about families, and they want the staff to understand the concepts behind a systemic way of working. We also recognize, however, that the staff is responsible for taking their clients through intake, planning, and subsequent procedures, and that all of this must be recorded on forms that enable the system to track what is happening. So, we have joined in this inevitable feature of the system by designing alternative forms, manuals, and procedures that not only cover the necessary ground but also convey a message consistent with a family-focused model. For instance, a new form for service planning, developed during the second project, highlights family issues and strengths, as well as specific goals and a time frame; a new form for observing visits between parents and child requires a record that is detailed, case specific, and cannot be filled in automatically; and the *Training Manual for Foster Parents*, which grew out of the first project, draws attention to facets of the foster care process that are not customarily dealt with, moving participants toward practical and realistic matters even as they absorb the underlying philosophy of the approach.

The orientation to concrete guidelines also takes the form of catchy phrases and slogans—a shorthand that is shared by the participants and reminds them of the basic ideas in the training. Just as the consultant in the adolescent residence for substance abusers (Chapter

5) kept reminding his group to "catch people doing something right," the consultant in the second project of this chapter developed phrases to help the workers deal openly with the mutual resentment that is inevitable between the families. He reiterated the necessity of "straight talk" in facing the realities of time and outcome, reminding the families that they "don't need to like each other, they just need to communicate." He also invoked certain "mantras" for the two sets of parents in their relationship with each other: "You have options; what do you think would be best for the child?" Simple tools of this kind help workers and parents to absorb and implement a new approach.

The Support of Social Policies

During the period of these projects, social policy was generally supportive of a family focus in foster care. Whatever the reality in actual practice, the stated aim was to reunite families as soon as that was safe and possible. The first project was clearly consistent with that goal and proceeded with reasonable social support. The situation was somewhat different when the second project was launched. A concern for the child's experience had become primary. Reunification of the biological family was still the preferred outcome but had become implicitly, or explicitly, secondary to the welfare of the child.

The mixture of policies that espoused a family orientation while emphasizing permanent solutions for the children provided both an opportunity and a challenge. The implied hierarchy of those two goals carried the danger that parental rights would be terminated early, in the effort to find a permanent home for the child. In developing the second project, however, the consultant saw this complex situation as an opportunity. He considered the two goals compatible and was able to formulate a multilevel intervention that would keep both facets at the forefront of the work. If consultants can integrate their programs and point of view with social policies, the possibility of creating enduring effects is improved.

There are no guarantees, of course, that social policy will continue to support particular interventions. Policies tend to be volatile, and new mandates may either negate the newly learned ways of working or undermine them by reorganizing the system and dissolving experienced teams. Whether the new ideas persist in any form depends on other factors, such as the duration of training, leadership, adaptability, the previous integration of procedures into the daily work, and so forth. If theory and training have been absorbed by personnel who remain with the system, the effects of a new program may be resilient, reappearing, in time, within the framework of different regimes.

Adaptability

There is no rest for a creative consultant or trainer. While the basic message never changes, circumstances and participants differ from place to place and from one period to another. The challenge is to adapt and reformulate in ways that can be accepted, while maintaining the core principles of what is being taught.

In the first foster care project, every agency required a particular approach toward administrators and personnel, even though the guidelines for training procedures were established, and the trainers needed to adapt to periods of challenge and discouragement within their training group—by stopping to review, returning to demonstrations, and taking their cues from those who were most resistant or confused as well as from leaders and enthusiasts. It is a task known to most good teachers, who must follow a curriculum but are constantly aware of who is learning what, and how they must adapt to the realities of their group.

While the necessity for adaptation was a recurrent experience for trainers in the first project, the clearest illustrations come from the later work. The formulation of the second project required a shift from staff training at specific agencies to consultation and demonstration across a broad spectrum of the foster care system. In the latter situations, it was necessary to relate to personnel carrying a variety of roles and to frame family-oriented ideas in ways that could be useful for their particular task.

Specific illustrations of flexibility in this work often took the form of suggestions or alternatives to routine procedures that are generally taken for granted. In one situation, the consultant questioned the automatic "cookie-cutter" approach of sending a mother and daughter to separate anger management groups to resolve their conflict, and the worker was then able to find a setting that would take them in together. In another, the consultant broke with the generally unquestioned protocol that was established in the hierarchy by going to the office of a law guardian who had blocked a process that was supported by other professionals. He knew that lawyers in that position do not meet with other parties, and that, barring further discussion, the law guardian's ruling would prevail. Following this break in the usual procedure, the problem could be resolved successfully. In other situations, the consultant brought workers back to a focus on decisions that were essential within the time frame of the case. In all these situations, consultants were modeling a flexible posture in dealing with situations that had well worn but nonproductive pathways, so they could make progress toward the goals.

Leadership Commitment

Commitment on the part of the leaders often appeared in combination with adaptability. Of course, creative leadership involves time, persistence, and the judicious exercise of power, but it also requires flexibility. In the evolution of the foster care projects, the ability of leaders to deal with system rigidities and to create alternatives in the face of problematic conditions was essential for supporting changes in policies and practices that would endure.

Intensive Family-Oriented Training and Supervision

Both the quality and duration of the training were essential elements in the effort to create enduring effects. Training during the first project was detailed and intensive, providing supervised hands-on experience with agency families and extending over a period of years in each agency. Most participants developed a family-oriented way of thinking about foster care and some skill in bringing members of the two families together for discussions and decisions concerning the child. We knew we had laid the groundwork for a systemic approach to foster care.

The major threat to continuation, aside from changes in policy, resided in turnover. Inevitably, the original cast of administrators, staff, and foster parents who had participated in the training project changed over time. As a safeguard for the continuation of what they had learned, it was essential for agencies to establish in-house structures: procedures and personnel to orient new staff to the agency's way of working; orientation sessions for new foster parents, to be conducted by those who had already been trained; and periodic staff meetings focused on peer supervision, the discussion of cases, and a consideration of how the basic principles of a systemic approach relate to new developments and administrative directives. One purpose of intensive training during the project was to create a staff with the competence and confidence to pass on what they had learned after the training had finished. The concepts and skills that are mastered in the course of careful training can only endure if they are reviewed and revitalized periodically.

Reflections on Integrating Family-Oriented Practices into a Large Service System

In the previous chapter, we identified an important factor in maintaining a family-based approach: the integration of family-oriented practices into an organization. It's important to note, however, that the scope of change is affected by the size of the system. When the target is very large and the new approach requires major shifts at multiple levels, interventions are not likely to create a lasting impact on the entire system. We have learned two important things from tackling foster care in one of the largest systems in the nation: Progress tends to be partial, and all the factors we can identify must probably be operative at the same time, if widespread changes are to take effect and endure.

Evidence of progress in affecting the foster care system appeared in many forms: in institutions that incorporated the family-oriented forms and procedures that had been developed; in agencies that established peer supervision for family work at the end of the project; in ripples created by alternatives presented to lawyers, judges, and other personnel from related fields who affect foster care decisions; and in requests for workshops, consultations, videotapes, manuals, new forms, and published material. It's not possible to say, however, that this, or any like-minded program, has shifted the vast foster care system to a comprehensive position consistent with a family-based model.

What does seem possible is that a combination of factors may, in the long run, be effective. If factors such as we have been identifying were all operative in the same situation, it seems possible that major positive changes could be created and sustained, even in relatively large and complex systems.

APPENDIX 6.1. TRAINING MANUAL FOR FOSTER PARENTS
BASED ON AN ECOLOGICAL PERSPECTIVE ON FOSTER CARE

Table of Contents

(continued)

Session Two: The Foster Child: Entering a New Home

To the Trainer (themes, skills, goals)
Session Activities
    I.   Child Development
    II. Connecting to the New Home
    III. Troubling Behavior: Understanding and Helping
    IV. Open Discussion

Session Three: Roots: The Foster Child's Biological Family

To the Trainer (themes, skills, goals)
Session Activities
    I.   Understanding the Biological Family
    II. Receiving Siblings into the Foster Family
    III. Open Discussion

Session Four: Different Kinds of Families:
Family Shapes and Ethnicity

To the Trainer (themes, skills, goals)
Session Activities
    I.   Family Shapes
    II. Ethnicity
    III. Open Discussion

Session Five: Visitation and Continuing Contact

To the Trainer (themes, skills, goals)
Session Activities
    I.   The Meaning of Visits and Family Contacts
    II. Encouraging Family Visits
    III. Visiting Time: Before, During, and After
    IV. Open Discussion

Session Six: Coordination with Case Workers:
Exploring Functions and New Roles

To the Trainer (themes, skills, goals)
Session Activities
    I.   Foster Care Activities in the Agency: Organized Services and New Roles
    II. Case Worker and Foster Family as a Team: Setting the Pace and Roles for Contact with the Natural Family
    III. Open Discussion
Appendix
       Sample Chart of Foster Care Activities

Session Seven: Coordination with Case Workers:
Implementing the Process

To the Trainer (themes, skills, goals)
Session Activities
  I.   Preparing for Contact
  II. Meeting with the Biological Family
  III. Solving Problems Cooperatively
  IV. Open Discussion

Session Eight: Going Home

To the Trainer (themes, skills, goals)
Session Activities
  I.   The "Going Home" Transition: Different Perspectives
  II. The "Going Home" Transition: Planning Together
  III. Leaving the Training

CHAPTER SEVEN

The Mental Health of Children

Jane has just turned 13. She sits at the window of the psychiatric ward, looking out. She's a little hunched over, drawn in, not responsive to the noise and activity of the children around her. She's waiting; maybe her aunt will visit today, and maybe one of her brothers or her kid sister will come along. Jane has been in the hospital for almost a year, but away from home since she was 9. She's been in three foster homes and in a residence for troubled and troublesome children. She's taken drugs, had outbursts that frightened the families she was living with, and has been diagnosed with depression. She was moved to this hospital because she was considered potentially suicidal.

In this chapter about the mental health of children and adolescents, we are not in new territory. There's considerable overlap with situations described in the chapters on substance abuse and foster care. Many of the children, like Jane, move from one service jurisdiction to another, and many of the issues discussed in this chapter will be familiar, especially in relation to service systems and particularly with respect to children from poor, multicrisis, minority families. Yet there are special features when the care of children comes under the rubric of mental health. For one thing, the medical profession is in charge of diagnosis and treatment. Medical personnel have special qualifications and high status, and it's rare for patients, families, or other staff members to question their judgments. For another, some of the manifestations associated with disturbance at the extremes of mental illness (e.g., hallucinations, dissociation, profound depression, suicide) are mysterious and frightening to many people, and families readily cede decisions and treatment to professionals when their children become part of this world. Finally, the increasing reliance on medication to control and cure symptoms reinforces the authority of physicians, who are clearly more knowledgeable about such matters than other service providers or families.

Looking broadly at current policies and practices in the area of mental health, we see an active field, in which the old and the new coexist, and where policies may shift unexpectedly as experience accumulates or new administrators take charge. Nonetheless, it's possible to identify two prominent streams on the national scene: the first is a traditional way of providing services to mental health patients, whether adults or children; and the second is a more comprehensive approach to providing systems of care, in what has been referred to as "the new community psychiatry" (Pumariega & Winters, 2003).

The traditional approach, like all efforts in this area, is dedicated to treating problems. To accomplish this, it follows a medical model, focusing on the individual as the carrier of symptoms, emphasizing the description and diagnosis of pathology, and organizing treatment via medication and other mental health services. There is a clear formula for what aspects of the case must be in the hands of qualified psychiatrists and what aspects may be handled by others. Systems of reimbursement by HMOs and insurance companies reinforce the boundary around the identified patient, as well as this treatment structure, and may shape the nature and timing of the treatment.

Proponents of "systems of care" take a different view. In her discussion, Stroul (2003) notes that the vision, the policies, and the mechanisms for providing services have moved on from the traditional model, which has proven too limited and not sufficiently effective. The newer approach includes community resources, the participation of families, and "wraparound" services—a structure in which child and family are part of the planning process, services are drawn from the natural and professional community, and treatment is tailored to the particular situation and needs of each case (see Burns & Goldman, 1998; VanDenBerg & Grealish, 1996). The aim is to increase the possibility of a positive outcome by including and empowering families and by integrating services in a meaningful way. Proponents of this approach include some child and adolescent psychiatrists, though there is some concern in this group that the usual procedures for implementing the model lessen the role of the psychiatrist.

In our work as consultants and trainers, we have seen both the traditional and more comprehensive models in action. When mental health services were traditionally structured, our primary job has been to help staff understand the value of including families. In situations where families were already included, our focus has been on improving the process in such areas as the assessment of children and families when they enter the system, the training and supervision of staff who are implementing services within these new structures, and the role of families in these procedures. Much of this chapter is devoted to our work in these areas.

It should be clear that we consider the inclusion of families in this second model to be a giant step forward. In our approach to assessment and treatment, however, we go beyond the matter of respecting the family's viewpoint and giving the family decision-making power. We see the family as a force for healing. The desired outcome in these situations is for the child to improve and for the family to be able to live together. Family life is about relationships, and we believe that a broadened approach to the mental health of children must include a concern for family interactions that perpetuate problems. Our approach, therefore, involves the collaborative effort of skillful professionals and family members to explore how the family functions and to reorganize the pattern of relationships, when necessary, on behalf of a positive outcome.

In this chapter, we describe some interventions that have followed from this orientation, as well as the systemic issues that have facilitated or impeded our efforts. We begin with a foray into the world of psychiatric institutions for children designated as mentally ill. Following that, we describe our collaboration with a statewide mental health system, during which we focused on the training of professional staff and on the assessment and treatment of families.

PSYCHIATRIC HOSPITALS AND WARDS

Traditional Structures and the Introduction of Families

In institutional settings, such as psychiatric hospitals, the walls are usually effective boundaries, and we know that efforts to change the structure will usually need to start with the basic points: that families are essential for healing, and that an exploration of family relationships is a necessary part of understanding the child and planning the treatment. For psychiatric staff trained in traditional methods and accustomed to established procedures, family interviews are often a journey into the unknown. Demonstrations of such interviews by our staff do not bring immediate change, but they tend to stir the waters, perturbing the situation in a constructive way and suggesting the possibility of an alternative approach, especially for practitioners not fully satisfied with prevailing methods and with the rate of success.

In this section, we present three cases, highlighting in particular the introduction of a family perspective into the more traditional procedures that have characterized diagnosis and treatment to that point. The first two cases concern young people hospitalized in psychiatric wards: a withdrawn adolescent of 18 and an impulsive boy of 10, each of whom has been hospitalized for some time. Called in to meet with the family, in settings where that is not customary, the consultant believes that the central question is whether these young patients will need to spend much of their early lives in such institutions or whether they and their families can be helped to create a viable situation at home. The exploration begins by meeting with the families while the child or adolescent is in the hospital.

The third case concerns a suicidal adolescent brought to the hospital for admission to the psychiatric ward. This case highlights the relevance of ethnic diversity and cultural realities in evaluating young people with psychological symptoms.

Three Illustrative Cases

JURGEN: A WITHDRAWN ADOLESCENT AND A PROTECTIVE FAMILY

Jurgen is 18. Because of behavior that is sometimes agitated, sometimes delusional, and sometimes withdrawn, he has been diagnosed with schizophrenia and has been hospitalized for long intervals over the last 3 years. In the hospital, he is generally passive; a shadowy presence on the ward, moving slowly through the simple routines of dressing, eating, and going to activities. He improves over time, but the staff is puzzled by the fact that when he goes home on visits he regresses; he sleeps a lot, avoids friends, and becomes increasingly agitated and withdrawn.

Jurgen is back in the hospital now, and when the administrators arrange to bring a family psychiatrist to the ward for some consultations, the staff suggests that he meet with this family. The consultant knows, as he enters the situation, that family meetings are rare in a psychiatric ward, and that when they happen they are usually focused on gathering information about the patient or discussing individual progress. The consultant's primary goal, therefore, is to help the staff understand that family patterns are intertwined with the behavior of their patient, and that working with the family is a necessary part of the healing process. At the same time, he wants to provide the family with some new perceptions of how they interact, as well as some sense that such meetings are meaningful for the well-being of their child.

Jurgen, his father, his mother, and his two siblings have now assembled for the meeting, and, as they enter the room, they reflect an easy informality, introducing themselves and finding seats. An observer might spot Jurgen as the most reserved, slightly wary member of the group, but his behavior is not abnormal. As the consultant makes his first general contacts, he notices that Jurgen's speech is slower than other members of the family and that, in a very friendly way, other people tend to finish his sentences for him.

As the opening contacts move along, the following interchange takes place. The consultant is talking with Jurgen's sister about her boyfriend. He turns to Jurgen.

CONSULTANT: Do you have a girlfriend?

JURGEN: No.

CONSULTANT: Do you know your sister's friend?

JURGEN: Yes.

CONSULTANT: What's his name?

JURGEN: Perry.

CONSULTANT: How old is Perry?

JURGEN: (*Hesitates a moment, and when his sister says, "19," he says, "Yeah."*)

CONSULTANT: She's helpful. She didn't wait till you asked; she volunteered. Is that something she does frequently?

JURGEN: Yeah.

CONSULTANT: So she takes your memory.

The consultant is developing an idea that this is a basic pattern in the family. He asks Jurgen who else is so helpful. Jurgen indicates that his mother is, and the latter says, "I'm overprotective." His father says he's also like that: "I remember, over the years . . . things he wanted to do, I did it for him." The consultant asks Jurgen if he thinks all that helpfulness is a problem, and then suggests he discuss it with his father.

The father and son are sitting at opposite ends of the family semicircle and the consultant suggests that Jurgen move over to sit next to his father. Jurgen disconnects the lapel microphone he's wearing, sits down next to his father, and then reconnects the apparatus, moving the wires out of the way. His father, who is leaning toward him, reaches over and rearranges the wires.

At this point, the consultant walks over to stand in front of them and says in a strong voice, "That's exactly what happens!"

CONSULTANT: (to Jurgen) You came, and your thing was like that (moving the wires), and did you see what your father did?

FATHER: (smiling) I corrected, I thought. . . .

CONSULTANT: (continuing to talk with Jurgen) He took your wire and he put it here. Why did he do that?

JURGEN: I don't know. I guess he . . .

FATHER: (still smiling, and talking over Jurgen) . . . minding your business.

Everybody laughs except the consultant, who ignores the comment and continues to look at Jurgen, who says, "He was trying to correct something, I guess."

CONSULTANT: Do you have two arms?

JURGEN: Yes.

CONSULTANT: Do you have two hands?

JURGEN: Yes.

CONSULTANT: (lifting Jurgen's arm) Does this arm finish in this hand? . . . At age 18 can you do that? Isn't it strange that he should do that as if you broke your hand?

JURGEN: Well, he does that a lot. He tries to do things for me.

CONSULTANT: How old do you think he thinks you are? 3? (pause) 4? 7? 12?

JURGEN: (*thoughtful*) Maybe 12.

CONSULTANT: Can you help him to let you grow up? . . . so he can let you use your two hands?

JURGEN: I don't see how.

CONSULTANT: If you don't help your father change, you will always have 10 thumbs and two left hands. You will always be incompetent.

Through the rest of the session, the consultant explores this theme with the family, highlighting their pattern of taking over for each other. The pattern moves around the family in various combinations, but it is most damaging to Jurgen, who loses his voice, his capacity to decide for himself, and his ability to act. With all the repetitions, underlined by the consultant as they occur, it becomes clear to the staff and to the family that the family's interaction with Jurgen, though motivated by love and concern, is immobilizing a withdrawn boy who accepts their interventions without a challenge.

The style of this consultant is relatively dramatic, but any consultant or therapist, using his or her own style, can create a different framework for the staff and family by employing the kind of interventions that have been discussed earlier in the book: highlighting *enactments* that bring habitual patterns to awareness (e.g., others are finishing Jurgen's sentences, or rearranging his wires); introducing *metaphors* that the family can remember and carry with them (e.g., "They take your memory," "They are your extra arms and hands"); reacting with *intensity* in order to focus attention on behavior that is taken for granted but must be recognized as damaging (e.g., saying forcefully "That's exactly what happens!").

The session has demonstrated that Jurgen can respond more actively. He may require outpatient treatment, but he could probably live at home and improve. The staff understands that the family would need help in changing their patterns of interaction; they would need to tolerate Jurgen's pace, give him space to act, and listen to what he has to say. The session has offered some metaphors to start off with; the family and the therapist would come up with others. If the staff can implement this process, the cost of treatment will go down—always an important consideration for the system—and the quality of life may go up for both patient and family.

MARK: AN ACTING-OUT 10-YEAR-OLD AND AN UNCERTAIN MOTHER

The second case involves a younger child, 10 years old, hospitalized when he was 8, and subsequently moved to a psychiatric ward. Mark is diagnosed as having ADD (attention deficit disorder), and is described as a child who acts out a lot and is difficult to manage. The consultant has been asked to meet with the staff, conduct a demonstration interview with the family, and then meet again with the staff for a discussion.

In this case, the prominence of medication is striking; it is the central aspect of treatment. In presenting the case before the session, the psychiatrist's report is focused on the medical cocktail, describing in detail how the mixture has changed several times and how each trial did or did not control Mark's behavior. Other staff members who work with Mark each day say little, and when a counselor comments on activities that Mark enjoys, it draws little attention. Mark as a particular kind of child, with specific strengths and interests, is not part of the picture.

The interview brings together Mark, his mother, his 12-year-old sister, Janice, and his aunt and her 8-year-old son. The consultant starts the session by asking Mark to describe his family. As Mark responds, the consultant evaluates his cognitive development and his ability to communicate: He judges him to be a child of normal intelligence who is able to respond appropriately in a one-to-one conversation, though there are signs of restlessness and some idiosyncratic language. He notes also that Mark is describing a family that's close and supportive of its members, and that Mark is still very much part of the group despite his years in the hospital.

The consultant moves on, then, to work with the family. The following excerpt highlights only the segment that explores the relationship between Mark and his mother, since the interchange with mother and son illustrates clearly what was different in this approach.

CONSULTANT: (*addressing the mother*) Why is Mark here? (*then, immediately, to Mark*) Why are you here, Mark?

MARK: Because I have problems.

CONSULTANT: Why are you here and Janice is not here?

MARK: Because she's better than me, right?

CONSULTANT: (*to Mark*) You should ask your Mother why you're here.

MARK: (*to the mother*) Why am I here?

MOTHER: Because you have a lot of problems with me, a lot of problems with school. (*to the consultant*) He just wants to do what he wants. (*to Mark*) You have a lot of problems with me. It really came to a point where I couldn't handle you being home.

CONSULTANT: It seems you're saying that he's here because you couldn't handle him.

MOTHER: That's one of the reasons.

CONSULTANT: (*lightly*) Why are *you* not here?

MOTHER: (*surprised, and laughing*) Why am *I* not here? I don't know about that.

CONSULTANT: Mark, what do you think of this idea? If Mommy can't handle you, she should be here.

MOTHER: (*to Mark*) You think I should be here?

MARK: No.

CONSULTANT: The fact is that Mark will be here for a long time if you can't handle him. So there are two reasons why he's here, and one of them is that you can't handle him. Are you ready to take him home?

MOTHER: He has improved in a lot of ways, but when he comes home on passes, he doesn't want to listen to me. He doesn't show respect. But sometimes . . . he has improved a lot.

CONSULTANT: I will ask you a strange question. You said that he has improved. Have you improved as well? It's a two-way street, isn't it? It deals with how you and Mark get along. As soon as you will be able to take care of him, they will release him. If your relationship changes, he will change. It's a different way of thinking, isn't it?

MOTHER: Yes, it is. . . . But I think you're right to the point, because it does have to do with me and him.

The consultant then asks the mother to talk with Mark.

MOTHER: (*to Mark*) I want you at home. When I put you in the hospital, I expected you to be in for 3 months. It's now 2 years. I want you home. You understand that? And I want that we should get along better.

Mark hides his face and doesn't respond. He looks disconnected from his mother and the scene.

CONSULTANT: (*to the mother*) Do something that helps Mark to listen to you.

MOTHER: (*addresses herself directly to Mark, asking him to sit looking at her, and repeats*) I want that you and I get along better together.

MARK: I want to go and play with Jody.

MOTHER: If you wait, the session will finish soon and you will have time to play with Jody.

MARK: OK, I'll wait.

The consultant gets up, shakes the mother's hand, and congratulates her for her effective handling of Mark. The session continues in this vein for another hour. The consultant focuses continuously on the mother's competence in handling Mark and highlights the moments of conflict resolution.

The organization of the session calls attention to the way this consultant approaches the core questions: Who is Mark? What is his context? How should treatment proceed? He used the first 15 minutes of the session to make contact with Mark. He explored the child's knowledge of his extended family, and, while they talked together, the consultant drew some diagnostic conclusions about Mark's level of intelligence, his capacity to concentrate, his way of connecting with strangers, his concept of self, and so on.

Beyond these general conclusions about Mark's capacities, the consultant looked at this child in context. He had spent 20% of his life—2 years—in a psychiatric ward, but he was also part of an extended family to which he was emotionally connected. His long sojourn in the hospital was reframed as a result of his mother's difficulty in handling him effectively rather than as simply a product of internal pathology.

With this new perception of the situation, the consultant could suggest that optimal treatment should involve the mother and other members of the family, and that planning should center on the process that would enable Mark to return home. As in the case of Jurgen and his family, treatment should not only stabilize Mark's behavior but also help the family reorganize their patterns of interaction. When Mark leaves the hospital, contact should continue through the transitional period until appropriate local services are established.

LILIANA: A SUICIDAL ADOLESCENT AND AN IMMIGRANT FAMILY

Liliana, 16, was brought to the psychiatric ward by her frightened parents after telling them she wanted to die and had taken a large dose of pills. The psychiatrist and psychologist who interviewed her were skillful and empathetic, and they spent time exploring her depression and sense of social isolation. They learned that Liliana felt imprisoned at home by her parents, who imposed rigid rules that cut her off from contact with other young people. From the perspective of individual pathology, it was not difficult to arrive at a clear DSM-IV (*Diagnostic and Statistical Manual of Mental Disorders, Fourth Edition*) diagnostic assessment. Liliana was a depressed, suicidal adolescent whose symptoms were an expression of impotent rage against her family.

After the case was presented to the consultant, he discussed the necessity of expanding the understanding of a family beyond the view that a despairing adolescent describes in an initial interview. It's always important to understand the context of a patient's behavior, but in this case it was essential to note that Liliana was part of an immigrant Latino family. To be relevant and helpful, the staff would need to explore the particular patterns of a family whose subculture and life circumstances were different from their own.

The consultant met with the family twice; first with Liliana and her mother and then with Liliana, both parents, and her older brother and sister. What emerged was the story of an immigrant family and its considerable difficulty in adjusting to this country after arriving from South America 5 years earlier. Their economic and social condition had spiraled downward. The father, who was reasonably successful in his own country, had difficulty finding a job, and, after short periods of work, was currently unemployed. The mother, who had a poor command of English and little confidence in using it, was cleaning offices to keep the family afloat. Like many immigrant families, this family was faced with a new language, the loss of friends and extended family, the challenge of supporting itself, the frightening reality of living in a neighborhood run by armed gangs, and the involvement of their children with peer groups whose lifestyles were unfamiliar.

Perhaps the most poignant aspect was that the pattern of relationships between generations characteristic of their own culture was not effective here. The older children, now in their 20s, had gone through a period of using drugs. The parents, concerned and despairing, were imposing strict rules on the youngest daughter in an attempt to forestall the kind of behavior they had seen in the older children. Liliana was caught between two worlds. Though loyal to her family, she still wanted friendship and a social life among her peers.

For the staff, these two sessions brought a new appreciation of the contributing factors in this case. Planned interventions moved from a focus on adolescent pathology to the complex issues raised by the ineffective attempts of concerned immigrant parents to protect their children. In their subsequent work, the staff encouraged discussion between Liliana and her parents concerning a workable balance between control and freedom, leading to the development of rules that would meet the parents' concern for safety while allowing Liliana the autonomy appropriate for a responsible teenager. The older siblings, now relatively settled, were useful mediators. They coached Liliana about reasonable activities, and they helped the parents to accept the distinction between delinquent, unacceptable behavior and the normal activities of American adolescents. The family was encouraged to look for social contacts and support in their own community, and, after some further sessions, Liliana was discharged. In this case, a family intervention at a point of crisis prevented a long-term hospitalization based on a psychiatric diagnosis. At the same time, the process helped an immigrant family find its way with increased confidence.

Established Procedures and the Prospects for Change

Hospitals are generally embedded in neighborhoods that are culturally and economically diverse, especially in urban centers, and it seems essential for staff members to carry an internalized map of the human territory outside the hospital. When children are brought to a psychiatric ward, it's important for the staff to know that the experience of immigrant families creates a schism between generations, which adolescents may find difficult to handle; that a child's silent withdrawal may be a characteristic mechanism in certain cultures, especially in the presence of unfamiliar authorities; and that explosive behavior may reflect resentment toward workers who represent the power of the official system. Since the diversity is not only ethnic but also social and economic, they need to realize, as well, that if they cannot locate the parents of a child from a poor area, the grandparents, godparents, siblings, or aunts may be the child's support, and may be able to clarify the circumstances of the child's behavior and the details of family relationships. A comprehensive approach requires not only the recognition of diversity but also an ability to work with families, as well as a willingness to establish contact with local services and informal resources while the child is still in the hospital.

The realities of American society in the 21st century suggest that this effort is not only necessary but timely. Hospitals are under pressure to move their patients along quickly, and the more rapid discharge of patients creates a moral responsibility to preserve the quality of care as patients are moved back to families and communities. The mandate for short hospital stays is motivated primarily by financial considerations, but it also has potential advantages for the treatment of disturbed children and youth. It motivates the psychiatric staff to evaluate, treat, and discharge their patients quickly from an essentially unnatural environment. If that is done well, it means that the staff will explore family patterns and mobilize external resources in order to support children like Jurgen and Mark as they move to a more familiar setting.

But the pitfalls are obvious. In some cases, the pressure may mean that the move is from hospital to a long-term residence, where youngsters tend to linger in a kind of limbo. In other cases, the effort may focus on using medication to control behavior as the most efficient path toward discharge. Exploring circumstances and working with the family is a more complicated process, and it takes longer.

At least three things are required, if a traditional psychiatric ward is to meet the requirements of short-term hospitalization without sacrificing the quality of care: an expansion of attitudes and goals, the creation of collaborative teams, and specific training in areas that have not previously been part of staff preparation.

From our point of view, the major requirement is to bring a family perspective into the thinking and work of the unit. Description of the process that brought families into a residential center for adolescent drug users is relevant here (Chapter 5), and the three cases presented in this section offer examples of demonstrations that help a staff to understand how families are involved in the patient's behavior and can be part of the treatment. As noted, however, the estab-

lishment of such an approach requires time, some staff reorganization, and some provision for ongoing consultation and training.

A family-oriented consultant would do well to start with a theoretical presentation for the total staff, which includes the major principles of systems thinking, concepts about family organization and
variations in different ethnic groups, the relevance of such ideas to
the presence of children in psychiatric wards, and the spectrum of
possibilities for treatment. Demonstrations of family interviews, followed by discussions with the whole group, concretize the theories
and illustrate the process. That's a beginning, and it's important for
creating a shared framework in the ward, but the work must be carried by teams that work on integrating these and other aspects into a
system of care that is comprehensive.

There are precedents among health care professionals for the
formation of teams that provide their patients with collaborative services, and, as time goes by, there are increasing efforts to help individuals and families cope with the implications of scientific advances
(Grimes, 2003; McDaniel, Campbell, & Seaburn, 1995; Miller,
McDaniel, Rolland, & Feetham, 2006). Proponents take a biopsychosocial view of health as their base, considering that the health
of any one member is intimately related to the family context. Teams
composed of physicians and specialists in family treatment work as a
unit, sharing information and expertise, and they offer a useful
model for psychiatric wards.

The desirable mix in psychiatric settings would include professionals who have expertise in treatment and medication; others who
understand neighborhood realities, have contact with the variety
of services available outside the hospital, and are experienced with
"wraparound" procedures; and still others who are specifically trained
to assess and work with families, both during the child's hospital stay
and during the period when child and family must adapt to the return
home. In the functioning of these teams, it is the shared nature of the
work that is important, rather than the technical mix of disciplines.

Staff members who work with families need specialized training
and supervision if they are to assess families competently and help
them change patterns that sustain their child's symptoms. A trained
family therapist may fill the function, becoming a full- or part-time
member of the department staff, but it is also possible to offer specialized training to members already on the staff who are particularly
interested in the systemic approach.

It seems likely that psychiatrists will be slower to respond to

such an offer than other professionals, since their training emphasizes the biological basis of the symptoms and the power of medication to alter behavior. Their participation is important, however, and
it is often advisable to arrange separate meetings for this group.
Given the opportunity to discuss their reactions to the approach and
to explore the relationship between family work, individual therapy,
and the control of symptoms through medication, they may well find
a role that is acceptable within a collaborative structure. The team
approach is not oriented toward changing the biological orientation
of psychiatrists nor toward ignoring the usefulness of medication.
Rather, it looks at this orientation as useful but partial, to be supple-
mented by a systemic view of children in context and an increase in
the permeability of hospital boundaries, so that information about
extended family, school, church, peer group, and community becomes part of the planning and treatment on the ward.

MENTAL HEALTH SYSTEMS

Psychiatric wards are always part of a broader rubric: a state- or city-
wide system that oversees not only psychiatric institutions but also a
variety of other services for people who require therapy. Within this
structure, the implementation of a comprehensive approach is most
likely to take hold in local settings. Sometimes, however, an exploration of change is sponsored by administrators at the upper echelons
of the bureaucracy, and the work we describe in this section is such a
case. Administrators of Child and Adolescent Services in the Department of Mental Health (DMH) of a large northeastern state were
interested in bringing a family perspective into their sector. As a
result, they invited our center to create a training program that
would change the orientation of the staff and improve their skills for
working with families.[1]

[1]We wish to thank the following administrators for their support during the project: Phyllis Hersch, Director of Policy, Planning, and Training, Division of
Child/Adolescent Services, DMH, who instigated the collaboration and encouraged us throughout; Joan Mikula, Assistant Commissioner for Child/Adolescent
Services, DMH; Gordon Harper, M.D., Medical Director, Child/Adolescent Services, DMH; and Julia Meehan, Director of Child/Adolescent Services, DMH
Southeastern Area, who has implemented and carried on the family-oriented
work.

Though they provided an open door, the task presented obstacles and risks. The policies and procedures of the department were like barnacles on a boat—the product of years of accumulated decisions piled on top of other procedures installed by previous administrators. It would be our task to change a system that had been built around the perceived needs of the child, as suggested by behavioral symptoms and the DSM diagnosis.

The long-term aim was to influence procedures across the state, but initial efforts have to begin in an area of reasonable size. This state was divided into several administrative regions, each one subdivided into a number of sites and including local agencies that provided services. Our first task was to select a region that offered the best possibility for success. We felt ourselves fortunate when we learned of a regional director who had given priority to community resources in her budget and was invested in keeping children out of residential institutions whenever possible. She would become our guide through the mined territory of the state system.

Over the course of the next several years, our teams worked intensively in this region and others, training case managers, clinical supervisors, and other personnel to work with families.[2] In presenting details of this work, we have selected the aspects that may be of most use to the personnel of other large-scale mental health systems. We discuss *the organization of the training experience*, summarizing the features we have found to be productive; *the training of case managers*, who function as the gatekeepers when a child is to enter the system; *the extended service system*, which includes the case manager, the family, and the providers of service; and, finally, *a summary of a newly developed assessment model*.

The Organization of the Training Experience

Certain principles were generally effective in setting up the training program and we were able to follow them in most settings. They are summarized below in relation to the composition of the training group, the nature and role of the training team, the pattern of a training day, and the advantages of training through induction.

---

[2]In addition to Salvador Minuchin, the following served as consultants and trainers in this project: Leonard Greenberg, Daniel Minuchin, Magalit Rabinovich, and Fran L. Smith.

The Composition of the Training Groups

When a system is large and complex, the formation of training groups involves decisions about size and the mix of personnel, as well as the frequency of meetings and the duration of the work with each group. Once we had decided on a geographical area, the groups were formed by following certain principles: Include personnel from different agencies in each group, so the effects of the training can spread, but bring in two people from each agency so they can reinforce each other when new ideas and procedures are brought back to their own center. Keep the groups small enough for intensive training but large enough for a mixture of issues and reactions to arise among the participants. Rotate the training meetings around the different sites, so that cases from a particular agency can be seen on their own grounds, extended staff from the host agency can observe the presentations and family sessions, and participants in the training can expand their understanding of the population and organization at other settings.

Two groups were formed in this first situation. The 10 participants in each group came from five agencies and they met every other week, rotating among the agencies throughout the training year. This organization worked well. Rotating among sites may be more difficult to arrange than mixing personnel or working out the pattern of timing, but in a large and varied system, it has advantages. The several agencies served similar clients but tended to work differently; some focused on collaborating with other providers, some primarily addressed the children, others had day-respite or residential facilities so that children could move from outpatient to residence to home without changing therapists, and so forth. At each agency, the group discussed with staff how services were implemented and how family sessions fit into the context of their work. As a result, participants developed a more open view of possibilities in their own agency and a broader understanding of the complex mental health system within which they worked.

The Nature and Role of the Training Team

In working with the DMH training groups, we generally followed a team approach. The fact that two trainers were working together allowed for flexibility in their roles. During a family session, for instance, one trainer could be available to join the agency worker and the family, serving as a support for the worker and demonstrating ways of opening up new avenues of exploration. The other trainer could remain with the group behind the observation mirror, commenting on what was happening in the session and discussing with the participants their thoughts and reactions.

The pros and cons of such a structure are similar to the issues of working alone with a family or as a therapeutic team. The decision involves personal preference, as well as practical and economic issues. When possible, however, the presence of two trainers is useful. The separation of roles during family sessions, as well as the interaction of the trainers during discussions, provides a richer experience for participants in the group.

The Pattern of a Training Day

The training day followed a particular pattern. As noted in an earlier chapter, this kind of regularity anchors the process and is reassuring for the participants. In the morning, one member of the agency team presented the history of a family in treatment and the family was then seen for a live session. In the afternoon, the second participant presented a recorded session with a different family. Discussions were interwoven throughout these procedures.

When the staff began to present cases, it was evident that the participants and trainers had different perspectives. The staff tended to present in a familiar format; they described the problems presented by the identified patient, how the worker saw the child's needs, and how the family was responding to the child. The trainers, however, had a broader internal checklist. They were interested in the history of the patient, but they were also listening for other details: the participation of different providers, the family organization and dynamics, the family's unwitting participation in maintaining the child's symptoms, and the involvement of different family members in repetitive patterns. The trainers were also tracking indicators of family strengths, the position of the worker in relation to the clients, and the worker's understanding of his or her own style of working with the family. It's not surprising that a staff overlooks most of these aspects at first. The purpose of the training is to expand their understanding of family organization and the complexities of the therapeutic process.

Family sessions, followed by discussion, are the primary teaching device for this purpose, but videotapes or DVDs of a session are important because they can be stopped at any point. Trainers can elicit comments about repetitive patterns and family strengths, and can ask, as well, about the worker's intentions: "What were you thinking at that moment?", "What were you trying to do?" The group can then enter to discuss the match between thoughts and interventions—what got in the way of implementing ideas, what other interventions were possible at a particular point, and what might have been most effective in changing the direction of the session.

Training through Induction

Training through induction is a method we have advocated throughout the book. Workers in the mental health system are facing clients every day, and if they are to deal helpfully with families, as well as individuals, they need to survive in the realities of a session. A general orientation to system ideas, principles of family organization, and theories of change is essential as a baseline, but for a working staff, trainers must tie their teaching to concrete material. For this group, theory arises most naturally from practice.

In this brief overview, we have presented some principles and details concerning the organization of training in a large mental health system, including the mix of participants, the function of a training team, the pattern of a training day, and the emphasis on case-based teaching and learning. We turn now to an account of our procedures in training an important group within the mental health system—case managers. Their orientation and decisions are powerful factors in determining the services that will be provided and the experience of child and family.

The Training of Case Managers

Case managers are middle management, and they function as "gatekeepers" in the mental health system. They are responsible for the assessment of children, their acceptance into the system, and the selection of agencies that will provide the care that their symptoms and diagnoses demand. Case managers are generally expected to consider all the details of a child's psychiatric history, accumulate evidence of abuse or other trauma, probe the incidence of disturbance in other family members, and so on—a litany of pathology, failure, and diagnosis that indicates whether and how a child will fit into the array of available services.

The DSM label, as the cornerstone of this review, militates against the utilization of the family as the focus of care. Rather, the focus is on the behavior and diagnosis of the child. It was against this background that we faced our task: We would be asking case managers to recognize that children are embedded in their families, and to understand that it's necessary to look at families both as a context that maintains the symptoms of the child *and* as a context of their healing.

Our consultation started with a polemic. The case managers saw us as people imposed on them by the administration. We would bring procedures that were new but not necessarily better, and would probably make their lives more difficult. They would be expected to implement new practices, and, in keeping with previous experience, those practices would be abandoned later in favor of yet other demands. We represented a temporary whim from above.

So we began our work, as we have done in other situations, by "joining" with the people in the trenches. In this endeavor, the initial dialogue was about the definition of the case managers' professional identity. They saw themselves as *administrative staff*, trained to assess children and match them with appropriate agencies that would provide care. We saw them as *clinicians*, who made astute evaluations of the context in which the children lived, were knowledgeable about family circumstances, and often bonded with families in a kind of therapeutic joining.

It was an interesting dialogue, in which we positioned ourselves as supportive challengers. We were questioning the self-perceptions of the case managers and supporting an increase in self-esteem. As against their fear of becoming overwhelmed by a completely new way of assessing children, we were suggesting a more exciting way of working and an advancement in their professional status. Perhaps we were most convincing because we believed what we were saying. To us, it was evident that case managers are constantly exercising clinical judgment. We wanted them to recognize what they were doing and to function in that role with knowledge and skill.

Acceptance of such an idea takes time, and putting it into practice is difficult. The case managers were leery of conducting family sessions *in vivo*, especially in front of an audience of their peers. Training proceeded, therefore, in the form of small steps:

1. The trainers presented tapes of cases they had conducted, modeling their openness to exposure even while they were illustrating procedures and discussing patterns of the family.
2. Case managers brought in families to be interviewed by a trainer. In the afternoon of the same day, the trainers and the group viewed recorded segments of the session and discussed the therapeutic techniques.
3. In time, case managers brought in a family and sat in the session. They did not participate, however, unless they were responding to a question or wanted to make a comment.
4. The case manager conducted a session with a family, but with the proviso that a trainer would come in as soon as requested.

The process offered protection and support, and the case managers became increasingly secure. It took almost half a year, however, before they were able to think of themselves as competent family interviewers.

As the training proceeded and participants began to interview families, the trainers took on their different roles. While one focused on observing the dynamics of the family, the other focused attention on the case manager's style of intervention; and while one emphasized the therapeutic strategies required by the family, the other focused on expanding the case manager's therapeutic repertoire so it would be available for a variety of cases. When the consultants disagreed on issues, they made a point of expanding the exploration of their disagreement. They were emphasizing the fact that there are multiple truths in the art and science of therapy, encouraging the case managers to voice disagreements and facilitating conversations among the group members about what they thought and why.

The following case illustrates the training process: the work of the case manager in charge of the family, the roles and activities of the trainers, the teaching about how to move the therapy along, and the discussions between participants and trainers.

The Case of Jody

Brina, the case manager, had met twice with Jody and her family, though this was the first time she had brought them to the training group. Now 13, Jody had begun attending school in such an on-and-off pattern that the school was threatening to expel her, and Brina had been trying to avoid a residential placement. The meeting included Jody's mother, Laura, who worked as a guard in a woman's prison; Jody's father, James, who was a probation officer; and Geri, Jody's 16-year-old sister.

THE FAMILY SESSION: INTERVENTIONS AND OBSERVATIONS

As the meeting begins, the family apologizes for arriving late. They explain that the problem was Jody, who spent so much time in the bathroom that everybody was delayed. Jody complains that the water in the shower was only a trickle. The father says he will fix it, the mother counters that the shower was OK when she used it, and Geri agrees with her mother.

Brina seems comfortable during this interchange, and for the first 10 minutes she tracks the conversation, asking questions to clarify the issues. One of the trainers, watching with the group, discusses the way Brina is handling the family. She is friendly, and the family clearly likes her. The trainer knows that this style of interviewing is typical of the case managers and is the product of the department's ideology. If the problem is the individual pathology of the identified patient, the parents are victims of an organic illness and deserve support. And if the job of the case manager is to match Jody's symptoms to an agency that provides expert management of her particular illness, Brina will function as an ally of the parents in finding a cure for Jody.

The other trainer is concentrating on the family, and he points out that something important is going on that the case manager is not attending to. The family is engaged in a repetitive pattern of never-ending conflict: Mother and Jody fight, Geri joins mother, father is neutral and stays out, and Jody finishes as the challenger and the scapegoat. The trainer is concerned that the focus remains essentially on Jody's pathology. He wants to expand the assessment by exploring the involvement of other family members in the maintenance of Jody's symptoms. He believes it's time to enter the session.

The participants know, by now, that there are several options, both for the case manager conducting the session and for the trainers. At times, case managers have run their sessions on their own; in other situations, the worker has invited the trainer in; and sometimes the observers have "pushed" the team to intervene. The options have proven useful. The case managers are comfortable, knowing that the trainers can rescue them. At the same time, they know that the emphasis is on the positive aspects of what they are doing. The discomfort of demonstrating ignorance in front of one's colleagues has been alleviated by one of the established rules for group discussion: A critical comment can be offered only if the observer provides an alternative suggestion that is viable and better.

One of the trainers enters the session and addresses Geri first. He asks if she has noticed how powerful Jody is, and says he's wondering how she can be more powerful than both her parents; after all, she's only 13.

As the trainer talks with Geri, the other trainer maintains a running commentary behind the one-way mirror. He points out that his colleague has introduced a major change in focus. Jody is described now as strong and willful, challenging parents who seem to be helpless. With this new focus, he has moved the issue from pathology to interpersonal transactions between the parents and their rebellious adolescent daughter. And by "gossiping" with Geri, as if the older sister were a neutral observer, the trainer has avoided entering into the conflict.

Geri says, "I don't know, but she's always fighting with mother. She doesn't go to school, and mother yells at her that she needs to go. But she doesn't, so she wins." The mother interrupts to say that she's in a bind. Jody has been diagnosed with posttraumatic stress disorder (PTSD), and she doesn't know how to handle her. If Jody is sick, as the psychiatrist says, she's afraid of making demands on her. The father comments that he thinks the problem is behavioral, and that they need to ask the school to find a special class for Jody.

The trainer behind the mirror says to the group that the issue of how parents handle the implications of a psychiatric diagnosis is important, but that they will discuss it later. Meanwhile, the mother is asking for direct help: "Tell us what to do. We need guidance. Would you suggest that we use physical strength?"

Now it's Geri who challenges her mother's way of controlling, and as she talks, she heats up, yelling at her mother and dismissing her with a gesture, saying there's no point because she doesn't ever listen to her. It's a repetition of the previous pattern of interchange between Jody and her mother, and, again, her father sits passively as if the storm doesn't affect him.

The trainer behind the mirror comments that the family is now in completely new territory. By encouraging members of the family to talk among themselves, the other trainer has created a "natural enactment" that clarifies the family patterns. The mother is challenged by her daughters and the father remains invisible. As observers, the group is *seeing* how Jody's symptoms are maintained.

The trainer inside the session continues to talk with the mother. "Laura, I'm concerned about you. You seem alone in your battle to save your family." Then, turning to the husband, he says, "I'm afraid she'll break. What can you do to help her?"

The focus has changed again. With Jody no longer the center of the problem, the mother has become the "identified patient" and the problems of the couple come to the fore. The second trainer points out to the group that his colleague is joining with the mother, challenging the father to be helpful. One of the basic sources of healing is the responsibility of family members to care for each other, and, as the case managers already understand, it's vital to elicit that impulse. The trainer is focused on the couple, but he is relating to them as *parents* who need to collaborate in order to help Jody.

As the session proceeds, the process of learning continues at the two locations. The case manager of the family is collaborating directly with the consultant; she is involved, as he is, in the family's stress, and is learning directly from his interventions. The other participants are in a more relaxed situation, observing two aspects of the session—the techniques of interviewing and the assessment of the family.

POSTSESSION DISCUSSION

The Case Manager's Approach. After the session, the group discusses the points that emerged during the interview. They start with the case manager's style of intervention, noting the positive way in which she joined the family; her ease of contact and support, her familiarity with events in the family's daily life, and her acceptance of absurdities like the shower incident. But they also note the negatives; because there was no exploration, there was no novelty. The questions of the case manager only served to expand on themes that were already familiar to all the participants. It was as if the case manager saw herself as a friendly supporter, wary of challenging the family's reality and vigilant about not seeming intrusive or disrespectful. This was still a familiar style among the case managers, and it triggered discussion, once again, about functioning as a clinician in order to help a family change.

The Trainer's Intervention. The group then discusses what the trainer did when he entered the session. He had moved the emphasis from Jody-as-patient to the powerless position of the mother, and from there to the husband's lack of support for his wife in her efforts to solve the family's problems. If they were to function effectively as parents, the husband would need to help her.

The steps in the intervention began with the older sister, Geri, as a designated observer of the family, and then moved to Jody's self-destructive power and the connection between Jody's behavior and Laura's sense of helplessness and depression. Only then was it time to challenge the husband/father in his "neutrality," which could now be labeled as an abandonment of his responsibility and a focus for constructive change.

Discussion of the intervention dealt with what is sometimes called "a stroke and a kick"—a technique that offers support and challenge simultaneously. The discussion also clarified the process through which Jody had been moved out of the spotlight, though the focus of the session remained tied to her healing; that focus was, after all, the primary definition of the case manager's job.

The Issue of the Diagnosis. The group then returned to a matter that arose in many cases: the power of the psychiatric diagnosis. An official diagnosis labels deviant behavior as part of an illness—an object of observation and treatment that should not be questioned. The existence of a diagnosis tends to loom large in the experience of most families, confusing the parents and leaving them feeling powerless. The label also registers with case managers as the central fact about the child or adolescent. Though the fact of the diagnosis cannot be avoided, in this or any situation, the team was trying to help the case managers see beyond the label and intervene more actively: to understand the participation of the family in maintaining problematic behavior; to realize that their own unquestioning support of family patterns made them unwitting accomplices; and to accept the importance of challenging the family's rigid cycles of stimulus and response.

The process of bringing in families, conducting sessions, and teaching case managers through observation and discussion continued through the training years. Sometimes the focus was on techniques, sometimes it was on family organization, and sometimes it was on issues that involved the larger service system; usually it was a mix. As time went on, the effort to extend a family orientation to the collaboration between case managers and service providers became a major factor in the training. Meetings that brought together providers, the case manager, the child, and the family represented a frontier—difficult, not always successful, but an opportunity for case managers to deal in a new way with the reality of the system around them. In the next section, we discuss the structure of this extended service system, and illustrate the effort to bring the relevant system together in a particular case.

Working with the Extended Service System

In the state where we were working, the treatment of children was delegated to approved agencies, known as "providers." When a child was referred to DMH, a case manager reviewed the case and then determined the assignment for services. Since each agency specialized in a particular area and was paid only for that function, the case managers referred children with multiple needs to a variety of agencies, with the result that treatment was frequently fragmented, redundant, and confusing. The case managers were the only professionals with a comprehensive view of the situation, and it was their task to organize and supervise the services of the agencies as well as the progress of the child.

As already noted, our training of case managers had emphasized the fact that their job required clinical judgment and an understanding of family systems. Once that basic fact was established, trainers could focus on the contact between case managers and service providers. The trainers maintained that the job of case managers was to extend the understanding of systems to the service providers, emphasizing the coordination of services in each case and communicating the importance of ensuring the family's involvement in treatment.

To serve that purpose, the group scheduled meetings that would include the case manager in charge of a particular case, the child and his or her family, representatives of the several agencies involved in providing services, and the consulting team. The remaining members of the training group observed through the one-way mirror, and the session was followed by discussion. What follows is a summary of such a meeting.

The Case of Ginger

THE FAMILY, THE SITUATION, AND THE HELPERS

The family consisted of 8-year-old Ginger and her mother, Sally, who was in her 30s and divorced. They were involved with both the Department of Social Services (DSS) and the DMH. A large cast of characters assembled for the meeting, including Ginger's teacher from first grade; the principal and teacher in her new school, which specialized in helping disturbed children; the case worker of social services, who was still involved with the family; the psychologist who was Ginger's individual therapist; the caseworker at the agency that provided respite when escalating conflicts exhausted both Sally and Ginger; and the case manager, consultants, and participants in the training project.

Before the family arrived, the case manager reviewed the essentials of the case: When Ginger was 5, there had been allegations of sexual abuse by a neighborhood adolescent. Ginger had periods of uncontrollable temper tantrums after that, during which she screamed and cried inconsolably. A psychiatrist had first prescribed Ritalin, and then a changing cocktail of medications. The symptoms persisted, and Sally asked the case manager to arrange hospitalization for Ginger.

THE FAMILY SESSION

The case manager brought Sally and Ginger into a nearby room while the assemblage observed through the mirror. During the session, the case manager and Sally focused on Sally's problems, paying no attention to Ginger, who had begun by moving around the room, then asked the case manager for some toys and settled down to play alone during the rest of the conversation. Sally poured out the tale of her difficulties in living with her daughter: Ginger didn't sleep, her behavior was erratic, and she cried whenever she didn't get what she wanted. Clearly, this was a mother under tremendous strain and a child who seemed not to draw attention when she was behaving appropriately.

POSTSESSION DISCUSSION

Case Manager, Mother, Training Group, and Providers Discuss the Case. After the session, the case manager and Sally joined the group of observers, while Ginger went into another room to play by herself. The discussion began with a recital of unending difficulties, described initially by the first-grade teacher, then the principal of the special school, the caseworker of the respite agency, the social worker from social services, the individual therapist, and finally by Ginger's mother. It was a competitive narrative of deviance: Ginger cut her hair and clothing with a scissors, she yelled and screamed, she hit other children.

One of the case managers from the training group asked if there was anything positive to say about Ginger. Basically a question about competence, it was a new way of looking at things that had been absorbed over time by participants in the group. It served as a challenge to the "healers," who had seen only pathology in the child, and the question remained in the air for a moment. Then the first-grade teacher said Ginger was creative, that she made friends with other children, and that she had long periods of functioning quite well. As if permission had now been granted, other people began to comment on positive aspects of Ginger's behavior. But Ginger's mother could not follow. She insisted that nobody had seen Ginger's behavior at home and that they were not aware of the extremes of her pathology. "If you experts don't know how to handle her," she said, "how do you expect me to succeed!"

Hesitantly, another case manager asked if there was something or somebody at home who might be provoking Ginger's tantrums. In that question, the consultants recognized, once again, the seed they had sown; it came from an understanding that behavior is interpersonal, and that parents and children are hooked into complementary responses. To everybody's surprise, Sally said, "Yes. Me!" Her patience was unraveling, and she was concerned that she might hurt Ginger if the child wasn't hospitalized for another assessment. The case manager hesitated, and then said she would make an appointment with the psychiatrist of the department. He would evaluate the situation, take a look at the current medication, and they would go from there. With that, the mother and daughter left and the rest remained for a debriefing.

The Case Managers, Consultants, and Providers Discuss the Case. The consultants began by focusing on the way that Ginger had been described. In a pileup of comments about pathology, participants had highlighted the behavior that confirmed Ginger's eligibility for services. The normal and competent aspects of her behavior had been described only after a case manager had raised a question about the positives—and it didn't hold up after the distraught mother returned to the problems she could not handle.

One of the consultants addressed the providers at this point, challenging their way of describing a child. His questions were expressed with intensity. "How could you see Ginger as a self-sufficient totality when we could all see the relationship between the behavior of Sally and the behavior of Ginger? . . . Did any of you think they needed to be seen together? And if you thought so, could you have referred them to a family therapist?" "Can you see yourselves, and the attitude of your agencies, as participants in maintaining Ginger's troubled behavior?"

As in a therapy session, a challenge expressed with intensity tends to startle the recipients, forcing them to look more closely at their assumptions and behavior. Reactions among the representatives of the agencies varied, but the message was clear for Ginger's case manager. After some thought, she said she would ask the psychiatrist to see mother and daughter together, would meet with the teacher to discuss ways of working with Ginger, and would help Sally to see Ginger as a complex child, with areas of skills and competence.

The Case Managers and Consulting Team Discuss the Role of the Providers. After agency representatives left the meeting, the group discussed the role of providers in this situation. Following the usual procedures, they had been offering a "hard sell" to Sally. There is a saying that "for a hammer, everything else becomes a nail," and, in this situation, each agency was suggesting to Sally that their services could straighten out the problems of her child. But such promises undermine the mother's sense of responsibility as a parent. The providers did not recognize the importance of the mother–daughter interaction; they did not attach importance to the fact that Sally was matching Ginger's tantrums with outbursts of her own, though Sally recognized the pattern herself; and they did not understand that services for Ginger alone, or even for Ginger and Sally treated separately, would not enable them eventually to live together in peace.

The Case Managers and Consultants Discuss Psychiatric Diagnoses. Finally, the group came back to the recurrent issue of how to work with the psychiatric diagnosis. It was necessary to accept the labels and admit their power, but it was also possible to expand the view of reality above and beyond what the labels implied. Meeting with Sally and Ginger together, the case manager could help them to develop less stressful, more adaptive patterns, using the resources of extended family, friends, and community as much as possible to support a more normal and satisfying life.

The Aftermath of Work with the Providers. Subsequent meetings with the multiple providers in a particular case followed a similar pattern. The meetings were useful, but they did not create a pervasive change in the system. In a structure where funding is channeled to particular agencies for the delivery of specific services, it's difficult to elicit cooperation rather than competition or to change ways of functioning that depower parents by taking over their responsibilities for caring, teaching, controlling, and healing. As one case manager commented, the prevailing approach is like that of a car mechanic: "You leave your car (or child) with me, and I'll call you when it's ready."

The usefulness of the meetings lay primarily in their effect on the case managers. As providers in different cases were assembled and issues of the case were discussed, case managers developed a broader, more detailed understanding of the larger system, and of the possibilities, as well as the difficulties, of their role. By the end of this intensive training project, case managers could approach their cases with a more systemic approach to the children and their families and additional skills for integrating and supervising case services. At least in a limited way, they could become agents of change for cases under their immediate control.

At the end of this chapter, we discuss the factors that have supported the survival of family-oriented work in some areas of this large and complex mental health system. In the next section, however, we offer a brief description of a family assessment technique developed recently by one of the authors (S. Minuchin). Because it is applicable to certain multicrisis families served by public systems, we describe the sequence of steps below and summarize the main features of an interview that followed this model. A full description of the model and of relevant cases is available in the volume by Minuchin, Nichols, and Lee (2007).

A Sequential Model for Family Assessment

We have maintained throughout the book that assessment must always involve the family, and have described the techniques of joining, enactment, intensity, and so forth that highlight a family's pattern of interaction and prepare the way for change. Excerpts such as those involving Jody, Ginger, and their families, as well as many others in previous chapters, illustrate how the process evolves in particular cases.

Though these detailed descriptions allow the worker to utilize the techniques effectively, the recent development of a four-step sequential model offers an additional guideline for the assessment process. Two new features of this model are particularly important: *description of the four-step sequence*; and *the exploration of past experiences that have shaped the way family members function in the present*. A clear sequence for initial contacts with a family is particularly useful for workers implementing a family approach for the first time, but it also helps experienced staff to stay grounded in the process and to move forward. Exploration of the past, which focuses on individual experience for part of the session, does so in the context of what has already been learned about current patterns of the family. Readers with some expertise in the theoretical basis of different approaches to treatment will note that this new feature combines a traditional interest in the effects of early experience with a more systemic concern for the forces that maintain current patterns of interaction.

We present the four steps briefly in the next section, followed by a summary of how the model has been applied to a family typical of the population we have featured in this book: a minority family, intermittently on welfare, whose multiple problems have come down through at least three generations, and whose lives are intertwined with a variety of service systems.

The Four Steps

The four steps are as follows: (1) opening up the problem and decentralizing the identified patient, (2) exploring for family patterns that maintain the problem, (3) clarifying the past experiences that have shaped restricted patterns in the present, and (4) working with the family on options for change.

STEP 1: OPENING UP THE PROBLEM AND DECENTRALIZING THE IDENTIFIED PATIENT

There is a basic question associated with this first step: *How can the family come to understand that the problem is broader than the official version, and that more people are involved than the identified patient?*

When young people are brought into the mental health system, the family takes it for granted that the problem is part of the child's internal dynamics, and the labels assigned by professional sources confirm their assumption. Bernard is described as a drug-abusing, acting-out adolescent; Chang as a deeply depressed and potentially suicidal youth; Myra as having a schizoid personality. All eyes are on the youngster, and The Problem, writ large, has become a summary of his or her identity.

It's the worker's task to challenge this perception; to create a broader, more three-dimensional understanding of this young person by drawing attention to areas of competence, reframing the problem, and replacing the stark diagnostic phrase with sentences that contain details and end in question marks. As this step moves along, the spotlight on a single individual dims and the ground is prepared for exploring family patterns.

STEP 2: EXPLORING FOR FAMILY PATTERNS THAT MAINTAIN THE PROBLEM

The basic question in this second step builds on the first: *What patterns in the dynamics of the family are contributing to the problem, and how can those patterns become visible to the family?*

Exploring family patterns is not a matter of identifying causes or assigning blame. Rather, it is a matter of exploring how family members, often desperate to help, are actually perpetuating a problem, repeatedly traveling in the same circles of interaction without recognizing that they are destructive. It is the worker's task during this step to bring the patterns to awareness as a prelude to change.

In fact, families often understand without too much difficulty that they are involved in the trouble. Jurgen's family came to understand that taking over his voice and his functions immobilized him rather than helping. Mark's mother was surprised at the idea that her helplessness was part of her child's lack of control, but found it believable and important. Liliana's parents could understand that the bewildering antisocial behavior of their children in this new culture had made them overprotective parents of their youngest daughter. It's important to explore these patterns without creating defensive reactions.

A variety of techniques for exploration are useful, but enactment, in particular, makes the patterns visible without imposing outside judgments. A family's typical way of relating to each other is almost sure to emerge during the session if the worker encourages the active participation of family members, and the pattern becomes part of a shared experience if the worker highlights its repetitive nature. The worker can also lead the family directly into a discussion, saying, for instance, "Let me ask you a strange question. How do you think the family is contributing to Randy's way of withdrawing?" . . . helping them past the first confused silence and encouraging the ideas that begin to come from family members.

This step should make it clear that family patterns are involved in maintaining the problems that have brought the child or adolescent into the system. The shift in perspective may be disconcerting for the family, but it also carries some hope; it implies that an effort to change the way they function as a family may alleviate the problems of their child.

STEP 3: CLARIFYING THE PAST EXPERIENCES THAT HAVE SHAPED RESTRICTED PATTERNS IN THE PRESENT

Here the question both opens up and limits a new exploration: *How were family members recruited, in the past, to see people and events in a particular way?*

This step explores the past as a way of clarifying the basis for current behavior, and it increases the possibility that current functioning can be expanded. Because this feature is relatively new, it does not appear in the examples described in this book, but it has been implemented in a variety of settings and has proven useful. It provides a way of understanding the forces that have restricted the patterns of relationship in the family and creates a more accepting atmosphere for exploring new pathways. Inquiries about the past are focused on the older generation—the generation in charge. The children are asked to be an audience, listening but not participating.

After a recurrent pattern has emerged in the family and the crucial role of a particular member has become clear, the worker might say, "It's clear that you want things to be perfect in your family, and that you take responsibility for making that happen. That must have started long ago. How did your parents make that such an important part of you?", or "We know now that you're expecting disaster to strike at any minute, especially when there are men around. The people who brought you up must have given you glasses for looking at the world that way. Let's talk about that."

The material that emerges is often dramatic, sometimes poignant, and it may surprise other family members, who have been asked to be present as silent observers. The atmosphere is often softer and more thoughtful at the end of this phase, especially if the earlier session has been characterized by conflict, and the family is often more willing to consider new ways of relating.

The worker must make choices during this step: who and how many people to interview (one or two adults are usually enough), whether all family members should be present or some sent out (if the children are young and the adult is reluctant to speak freely), and when to bring this phase to a close (when the influence of the past on restricting present behavior has become clear and further exploration would distract from the purpose of the session).

STEP 4: WORKING WITH THE FAMILY ON OPTIONS FOR CHANGE

Here the basic question is simple: *Where should the family go from here?*

This part of the model is similar to the process that finishes any assessment interview: The worker and the family draw together what has emerged during the session and discuss the implications for the future. No family leaves a session like this with the same view of the problem they came in with, nor do they have the same assumptions about how their family functions and what their role might be in the treatment of their child. For the family, then, this last phase is a matter of struggling to assimilate what they have learned, raising questions, and participating in a consideration of options. For the worker, it is a matter of summarizing the points that a family should carry away and leading a discussion of options that includes a new view of the family and a plan that is mutually acceptable. It's important, also, to finish by conveying a message of encouragement, support, and hope.

The Wilsons: Applying the Four-Step Sequential Model

Three generations of the Wilson family attend the assessment session: the grandmother, Sara, who is 52; her daughter, Sheila, who is 30; and Sheila's daughter, Kamisha, who is 15. Kamisha is living with her grandmother. She was removed from Sheila's care 3 years earlier by DSS, which declared Sheila an unfit mother, and Sara is now her legal guardian. Sheila is allowed to visit only under Sara's supervision.

Kamisha is 7 months pregnant and is receiving services from DMH, which has included her in a program for pregnant adolescents. Now, in the last weeks before the baby is born, decisions about the future are at a stalemate. Sara feels she's too stressed and too old to take on the care of a new baby. Sheila, who has finished a training course and started a new job, says she can't help out. In any case, DSS has indicated that Sheila cannot be in charge, and that the children should remain with Sara.

The family has been sent for an assessment, and the consultant who sees them will be following the four-step model in gathering information and working with the family. We present a brief summary of each step in the sequence, as applied to the Wilson family, and refer interested readers to the volume by Minuchin et al. (2007) for a fuller account of the process and verbatim details.

STEP 1: OPENING UP THE PROBLEM

From the narrow perspective of the service system, Sheila's behavior is seen as the problem. However, the consultant goes into the session knowing that the situation is much more complex—partly on the basis of the little he knows about this family but mostly on the basis of what he knows about the experience of families like this in society and with the service systems. The problems are social and organizational, as well as specific. They involve the burdens and tensions of three-generational matriarchal families, erratic relationships between men and women, the repetitive cycle of teenage pregnancies, the complexities of kinship foster care, the overall aura of poverty, and the resulting dependence on large public systems.

With all this in mind, the consultant begins by asking the family how *they* see the situation. The grandmother responds first. She's forceful and articulate, but as she talks about Sheila, her comments switch back and forth, indicating her needs and her ambivalence. She says first that her daughter is capable of taking over the parenting role, then that she doesn't believe Sheila will do that, and then again that it's really time because she, Sara, is tired.

When Sara moves onto the problem of her granddaughter's pregnancy, she talks as somebody who's "been there." She tells Kamisha that she will have a lot of hard things to endure, and that she will end up disappointed in her boyfriend. It's clear that Kamisha and Sara are close, but it's also evident that Kamisha resents her grandmother's predictions.

The consultant sees that there's tension between Sheila and Kamisha, and he asks them to talk together about the current situation. Sheila is gentler with Kamisha than Sara has been, but Kamisha pushes her off impatiently. She says she can talk about herself with her grandmother but not with her mother.

As this first step proceeds, it becomes clear that all the family members are involved in the problems, and that the issues carry emotion and create conflict. What has emerged is Sara's strong role, with its mix of entrenched control and resentment; the coalition between Kamisha and Sara; the barrier that blocks Sheila from helping out, arising not only from the rulings of DSS but also from within the family and, perhaps, herself; and the messages that pass, unheard in both directions, between the female adults who have "been there," to their wisdom and sorrow, and the more naïve and hopeful pregnant adolescent. The consultant says that it's important to explore the patterns that are making solutions so difficult.

STEP 2: EXPLORING FOR FAMILY PATTERNS THAT MAINTAIN THE PROBLEM

The consultant understands that separating children from parents and placing them with a grandparent in kinship care always complicates a relationship that may already be tense. He begins this part of the session, therefore by asking both adults why Kamisha has been living with Sara for 3 years. Sheila's version is that circumstances piled up: When Kamisha's father left, she had no child support and needed to work, but when DSS learned that the child was sometimes left alone, they took her away and appointed Sara as her legal guardian.

Sara's version is that Sheila moved out of the house when she became pregnant and has refused, over the years, to stay in contact. She claims that Sheila prefers the freedom of being on her own to taking care of her daughter, and that it has been hard on Kamisha. The two women go around in circles as they talk: Sara is critical, predicting failure, and Sheila is defensive, claiming she tries to change things but doesn't get anywhere. Their interchange is painful for both.

The consultant highlights the pattern, and says they will need to turn to the past in order to understand the roots of the behavior that is creating so much trouble: Sara's intransigent sense of responsibility and Sheila's tendency to act against her own best interests, as well as Kamisha's lack of trust in what adults, particularly her mother, have to tell her.

STEP 3: CLARIFYING PAST EXPERIENCES THAT HAVE SHAPED RESTRICTED PATTERNS IN THE PRESENT

Exploration of the past brings up dramatic material. In response to the question of how she became so overly responsible, Sara says it was because her alcoholic mother "didn't do her job." As Sara describes taking care of her younger siblings from early childhood on, the consultant comments that Sara "grew up in a box," with little freedom to relax or explore. He has created a metaphor that will be useful throughout the session.

When Sheila talks about her childhood, she says that she grew up knowing she was less favored in the family than her sister because she had darker skin. People teased her about it, and she was rejected by her grandmother. She says she was so hurt and resentful that she began to "do bad things." Sara is shocked, saying she was never aware that Sheila had such feelings, and she doesn't quite believe it. She thinks maybe it was just a sibling thing. Sheila challenges her, in tears, providing details from childhood experiences. Their interchange is intense, opening up the deep roots behind their mutual lack of trust.

When Kamisha responds to questions about her early childhood, she talks about the way her father treated her mother and about her fear of the violence. She doesn't talk directly about her sense that her mother abandoned her, but she says that she has never been able to trust Sheila or tell her things, and that she hasn't wanted to live with her because she doesn't like her mother's friends. Sheila tells Kamisha that she loves her but finds it hard to talk with her, and that she backs off a lot because Kamisha criticizes her so much and that hurts her.

At this point, the consultant knows that a lot of the past has been opened up, and that not only he but also the family members understand more clearly now where the repetitive and destructive behavior has come from. The family knows it must change, but they are caught in a family dynamic that has crystallized. They don't know how to break the vicious cycle of their interactions. The consultant says it's time for the family to consider their current options.

STEP 4: WORKING WITH THE FAMILY ON OPTIONS FOR CHANGE

The consultant asks the family what shape they want for the future. They all agree that they need each other's help, but the consultant says they will need to work on their usual patterns, which are continuously critical and convey little trust. As he sums up, he emphasizes the fact that Sara always thinks she can handle everything, even though she resents it, but it isn't true. She can't manage it anymore. In a major shift from the way the family and the service systems have been thinking and acting, the consultant addresses himself to Sheila. He says that her mother can't get out of the box by herself and that Sheila will need to help. He is drawing on his conviction that family members care about each other, and that they respond to the responsibility of helping the people they care about. He is portraying Sara, now, as the family member who needs help, and Sheila as the one who can heal her mother.

The consultant has assessed this family as caught in repetitive circles of attack and defense. They need but don't trust each other; they want support but push it off. He says they will have to ease the burden on Sara, as they work with their therapist, and that the roles of both Sheila and Sara must change.

There was a short follow-up to this assessment. The therapist working with the family reported that all the participants were angry during the next session, but by the second week, Kamisha had moved to Sheila's house. A month later they were exploring how to tear the "box" and working on the multiple problems that never go away, for this population, but that can hopefully be handled with less conflict and pain.

The case is not just the saga of these three women. We have summarized the session here not only because it illustrates the four-step model but also because it describes the conditions that exist in the culture of poverty: the relationship formed between men who take on too little family responsibility, for a host of reasons, and women who shoulder too much, depending on each other and coping as best they can. It also involves, in no small measure, what has been referred to in an earlier chapter as "the cookie cutter approach," in which system providers create separations and solutions without sufficient information or thought, thereby creating needless damage and compounding the problems of their clients.

WHAT ENABLES A NEW APPROACH TO SURVIVE?

As we come to the end of the chapter and address the question again of what enables an approach to survive, we limit discussion to our interventions in the mental health system of the state. Brief demonstrations, such as the family sessions presented in the first section of the chapter, have no clear subsequent history. They are seeds dropped into a field, and the effort is worthwhile simply because the seeds may take root; the ground may be unexpectedly fertile, or one or more "tillers of the soil" may find the new mix so interesting that they begin to think or function differently. We have no clues, however, about when, how, or why that happens.

The training project with DMH was much more extensive. Here we can look for evidence of change, and for the forces that enabled new, family-based practices to continue. We understood from the beginning that the effects could not be pervasive. Working with a statewide system of mental health is similar to the experience of working with a foster care system in a major metropolis (see Chapter 6). Comprehensive enterprises such as these are administered through many different agencies, employ many people, and carry out their functions through an entrenched bureaucracy. Though we were invited to bring a family-centered approach into the department, there were areas we were not involved in, such as the division of adult services, and procedures we could not touch. As in the foster care system, the impact would necessarily be partial.

Nonetheless, we had access to the division of children and adolescents, we were able to concentrate on settings where the administrators were strongly supportive, and we knew that our mission was important. We created positive changes that have persisted over time, and there's reason to expect that the effects may spread further, as circumstances change. A decade after our original foster care project, for instance, the top administration became more identified with a family perspective than we could have foreseen when we entered with our initial challenge. The effort to identify factors that maintain the vision and details of a family orientation is useful and important, even in relation to a large bureaucracy that resists the introduction of change.

The relevant factors in the area of mental health are similar to those that have emerged in the previous chapters:

- Intensive family-oriented training and supervision.
- Integration into organizational policies and procedures.
- Leadership commitment.

Intensive Family-Oriented Training and Supervision

The intensity, quality, and duration of the training emerged, again, as an important factor. In the meetings conducted by our teams, the experience for participants included demonstrations of family sessions, direct supervision of their contact with clients and families, discussions of theory and technique that arose from case material, and the kind of focus on the strengths and blind spots of individual workers that is possible only in small groups. All of this is essential for preparing practitioners who can function with confidence, skill, and sensitivity.

The appropriate duration of a training project is a difficult matter to decide. How extended must training be in order to make the investment of time and funds worthwhile; that is, to create an enduring capacity among the participants to continue on their own? Working well with families is a complex matter and the training takes time. It's important to note that a family-centered way of working has endured most successfully on the sites where the training continued for 3 years. In that region, groups continued to meet for case discussion and peer supervision after the project finished.

The latter fact is important. If the learning is to be strengthened, continuing review and supervision is essential. The original training is the core, but theory and practice are most likely to survive if they are periodically reinforced. Supervision should become an ongoing enterprise. It may be conducted by institutional staff who have been thoroughly trained in the new approach or it may take place through periodic contacts with outside supervisors. Both structures have appeared on the sites involved in the project.

Supervisory groups have a number of functions, some acknowledged as part of the agenda, others more subtle. The participants review cases, troubleshoot when a family presents a difficult problem, handle the erosion of a common perspective by orienting new workers, discuss how to integrate their approach with new policies that come down from the administration, and maintain their sense of purpose through the shared beliefs and experiences of the group.

In areas where the training was interrupted after a shorter period, the effects have been variable, but a family orientation has persisted on sites where the participants and the trainer were motivated to continue their work. One consultant responded to the needs and interests of her groups by volunteering time when funding was no longer available—much as the consultant working with drug-dependent women had done in a similar situation (see Chapter 5). In both situations, some funding subsequently became available and the groups were able to contract for additional periods of regularly scheduled supervision. The establishment of a structure for continuing in-house supervision is a more stable and desirable way of solidifying what has been learned, but, in the absence of such arrangements, some groups have found informal procedures for continuing their contacts and maintaining their family orientation.

No training project can inoculate participants with what they will need in the future to continue the work. A training project conducted by outside experts must be transformed, over time, into a different, renewable form. Optimally, ongoing training will be conducted by staff members who have integrated the new procedures into their way of thinking and working, but it is also possible to follow different procedures, as long as they monitor erosion, continue to refresh and develop staff skills, and are scheduled periodically.

Integration into Organizational Policies and Procedures

In the section of the state where the training had the most consistent support and lasted the longest, features of a family-oriented infrastructure have been established. Family-based practices have become "the way things are done," and in a bureaucratic system, that is the key to the survival of a procedure.

On these sites, new staff receive a basic orientation centered on children and family systems, case managers are supervised weekly and attend monthly meetings that reinforce a family perspective, and the staff has organized ongoing discussion groups or arranged contracts that bring in consultants to supervise the work with families. We remind ourselves and the reader that these are partial gains, but to the extent that they are integrated into the system, they are a clear step forward. They serve as the basis for further innovations, if and when the conditions are supportive.

As we have noted earlier, one way to ensure the adherence of staff to a new way of working is through the availability of concrete family-oriented guidelines and materials. It's not easy to change forms and procedures that carry the imprimatur of top administration and are followed throughout the system, but it is sometimes possible. One interesting example concerns the forms used throughout DMH when an applicant is considered for entry into the system. The statewide "comprehensive assessment" forms are long, detailed, and essentially focused on the individual applicant. In at least one area of the child-and-adolescent section, however, the forms have been modified so that they are more relevant to a family-focused approach. They now contain "areas to explore," following standard questions, requiring the worker to provide more in-depth information. Known as "prompts," these additions keep the family of the child or adolescent front and center, as the case manager considers needs and resources.

Consider the following examples: Case managers must summarize the problems that require DMH intervention and review the client's assets. The "prompts" that have been added for this item call for particular details, such as the parent(s)' kinship network and support system, their use of resources to assist them in parenting, their patterns of problem solving, and their sense of hope. Another item requires a psychiatric and psychosocial history, and stipulates specific details concerning illness, treatment, placements, hospitalization, and so forth. The "prompt" that has been added takes a different perspective. The case manager is asked to include a description of such characteristics as family roles, boundaries, power relationships, response to significant life changes, and rigidity versus flexibility. When the treatment plan is to be described, the "prompt" asks about the inclusion of family members in the planning, and when an item asks simply whether the parents are married, separated, divorced, or deceased, the "prompt" asks the case manager to evaluate and describe each parent's ability to meet the child's basic needs and provide appropriate supervision, as well as about the methods of discipline the parent tends to use.

Modifications of this kind are powerful. They shape the way staff members think about a case, and they determine the procedures through which a worker includes and relates to a family. Such concrete changes also illustrate a very important principle: It's possible, at times, to work within the boundaries of mandated forms and procedures while adding emphases, categories, or details that express a different perspective. If one cannot dispense with traditional procedures—and we sometimes could not—a modified tool may provide richer information than the one in use and come closer to the goals one values.

Leadership Commitment

The commitment of DMH administrators was crucial for our work. While the interest of an executive staff is not sufficient to produce widespread acceptance of a new approach, little can go forward without approval from above. Our work on the original sites profited greatly from the atmosphere created by the director of the area and the practical moves she initiated, and we were able to extend the family-oriented training into new areas, after the first phase, because department administrators were helpful in organizing the extended program.

During the early stages of training, the presence and approval of administrators is reassuring for staff as they face a demand for change. At later stages, executive authority is necessary for the resolution of issues that arise and for implementing decisions that have been agreed upon. Some of these issues are simple and relatively local, such as the provision of space and time for meetings and supervisory sessions, while others involve departmental matters, such as partial revision of the assessment form to include family material, a review of the fit between new procedures and union specifications, or integration of the wraparound approach with other conceptions of family-focused work. At times, the input of the administration on behalf of a family orientation has involved the power of the purse; for example, department funds have been used to cover aspects of the therapeutic work that are not recognized or reimbursed by insurers. Such details, initiated or approved by administrators, support the survival of the new procedures.

The commitment of administrators comes basically from themselves—from their interest in the approach and their willingness to use energy, skill, and influence in supporting the continuation of the work. But it's worth raising the question of whether and how that commitment can be mobilized when we enter a system to teach a new set of ideas and a new way of working. We consider that question, among others, in the final chapter.

CHAPTER EIGHT

Moving Mountains

Toward a Family Orientation in Service Systems

Over the past decades, our work within helping systems has expressed a consistent philosophy: the belief that a systemic, family-oriented approach to service is the most effective, economic, and humane way to work with people in need. Like all proponents of a new way of working, we have not always been able to create a lasting impact, but we have seen evidence of long-term effects in many situations; that is, the persistence of a family-oriented way of thinking and a systemic way of working still present in a variety of settings after a period of years.

What accounts for the positive effects? Why have the philosophy and practices of this approach taken hold, in certain places, despite the inevitable pull of forces that encourage regression to what has been standard and familiar? Because that is such an important question, we have carried it as a central theme in this edition of the book. After describing our interventions in relation to substance abuse, foster care, and the mental health of children, we have tracked the continuation of family-oriented services over subsequent years and considered the question, in each area, of what factors enabled this approach to survive.

As a result, we can now indicate the defining elements of a family-oriented service system and summarize the factors that contribute to their establishment and endurance. In Table 8.1, the defin-

TABLE 8.1. A Family-Oriented Service System: Defining Elements and Factors That Support Survival

Defining Elements	Relevant Factors
Skillful Practitioners of Family-Based Services	• **Family-Oriented Training:** Intensive training and supervision that extends over time
	• **Available Tools and Procedures:** Concrete family-oriented guidelines for the use of staff
	• **Systemic Orientation:** An emphasis on recognizing systemic structures and connecting system elements for contact and communication
Consistent Family-Oriented Procedures within the Organization	• **Integration of the Approach into Institutional Procedures:** The absorption of family-oriented practices into the ongoing work
	• **Leadership Commitment:** The activities of administrators and other leaders supporting a family approach
	• **Stakeholder Involvement:** The mobilization and investment of service recipients and staff in family-oriented services
	• **Adaptability:** The ability to adapt to local realities and changing conditions without compromising basic principles
Social Support for Family-Oriented Practices	• **Social Policies:** A framework of ideology, practical regulations, and available funding that supports a family-based approach to service

ing elements are listed on the left and the factors that are relevant for creating and supporting each element are listed on the right.

It has only been possible to construct such a list after considerable experience and the passage of time. We did not conduct our interventions over the years with such guidelines in mind. It's probable that our trainers were aware, at some level, of the forces that mattered, but they were necessarily focused on the immediate tasks that kept them busy: conveying the value of the basic philosophy, formulating the procedures that turn ideas into practice, adapting to the characteristics of different settings, and so forth. It's only now, after multiple interventions and a process of review, that we can track the features that have led to desirable changes and that appear to sustain them over time. To know such things in advance, of course, is an advantage. Perhaps the reader can think of the list as the contents of an intervener's pouch, providing useful guidelines for planning what to do and for evaluating how things are going.

In the remainder of the chapter, we present an integrated summary of the factors that maintain the basic elements of family-based services.

SKILLFUL PRACTITIONERS OF FAMILY-BASED SERVICES

A systemic family orientation can survive only if there are competent practitioners to carry it forward. The creation of such a group depends on training, the availability of relevant tools and procedures for the use of the workers, and the development of the staff's ability to understand and implement systemic connections.

The skill and confidence to implement such a role depends, first and foremost, on training. The nature of our *intensive supervised training* has been described throughout the book. We have presented a way of thinking that places the individual in a broad context and have described the skills that must be mastered for working with a family. Some of the skills are relatively easy to learn. Once described and illustrated, it's not difficult to map a family system, and for workers in the helping professions, it's often second nature to "join" a family by acknowledging their perspective and supporting them in their troubles. Other skills are more difficult, however, either because they're unfamiliar, such as the creation of "enactments" that illuminate family patterns, or because they're uncomfortable, such as challenging accepted family patterns or dealing with conflict. As must be evident in the examples and case discussions, however, a skillful practitioner is necessarily involved in supporting, challenging, and exploring alternatives, often at the same time, and the ability to do that requires repeated and varied experiences over an extended period.

As any experienced educator knows, it's important to offer new material in several different ways. In our training procedures, we present the fundamental concepts and techniques for working with families using multiple media: demonstrations, lectures, recorded family sessions that can be stopped and reviewed, supervised hands-on experience in sessions with agency families, and small group discussions. How long is "enough" for such a training process? That's difficult to say, but it cannot be accidental that in the settings where trainers were present for 3 years, the impact of the training was clearest and most sustained.

Intensive basic training is essential, but it may not be sufficient, in itself, to support the continuing practice of family-oriented services. Changing policies, organizational pressures, and the entrance of new workers into the system make it difficult to maintain such nontraditional procedures. We have come to understand that the persistence of a complex approach depends on a process that occurs in two phases: an *intensive period* of reasonable duration during which experienced trainers teach and supervise the staff, and a *continuing program* that is less intensive but that organizes review and case supervision as part of the staff's experience after the original training has finished. A Chinese leader once commented that each generation must reinvent the revolution, and that axiom is probably applicable to most organizations. Continuing discussion, as time goes by, allows a working group to own and develop what they have learned from their predecessors.

Programs that refresh and extend the learning have been established in a number of places, and they have taken two forms. In some settings, the creation of stable structures within the organization provides for a continuing process of in-house training. The activities are usually supervised by members of the staff who have become proficient during the initial training, and include regularly scheduled meetings for case reviews, orientation of new personnel, peer supervision, and consideration of how to maintain a family orientation while adapting to shifts in system regulations.

Procedures that have become part of the organization in this way are probably the most effective, but less stable forms of review have also been implemented and they serve the same purpose. Using outside supervisors, discretionary funds, informal structures, and irregular scheduling, interested agencies have also found it possible to sustain a family orientation and have been able to advance the relevant skills of their staff.

The creation of concrete *family-oriented tools and procedures* for staff use has emerged as a second factor, supporting the development of competent practitioners and reinforcing their continued implementation of a family-based approach.

Standard forms are part of most responsible organizations but they are particularly prevalent in the public sector, where there are concerns about the accountability of staff and the tracking of cases. In large service systems, forms and procedures are almost always oriented toward the individual, with a particular emphasis on the pathology deemed to require attention. There's an implicit message in this material, and the assumptions become ingrained in the staff through daily use. If workers are to maintain a family-oriented perspective, they must be offered concrete material that highlights relationships, the context of the individual, and indicators of strength.

It's not so difficult to create procedures of this kind to guide the way information is gathered and staff members relate to their clients. We have offered examples throughout the chapters. Some are focused on the initial contact that takes place when clients enter an agency, such as procedures for assembling family members, a form to guide questions about relationships, or a sequenced model for assessing family patterns and exploring alternatives. We have also created a manual for training foster families that has been widely distributed, and have designed time-bound and goal-directed forms for planning the steps in foster care cases and describing the visits between birth parents and their children, so that the case can progress without getting bogged down. In some instances, we have simply suggested that a staff revise their procedures to include family members, and they have proceeded on their own; a case in point is the process developed by staff members for consulting parents when decisions must be made about adolescents living at a treatment center.

Materials that express a point of view can be created and codified by any group that brings a new way of working to the staff of an institution. However, such tools should not be used rigidly; rather, they should serve as useful leads into important territory and should be modified as required by local conditions and particular cases. Because they organize the scope and content of staff contact with their clients, however, they consolidate new learning, and they reinforce the probability that the implementation of family-based practices will continue beyond the period of training.

What is more problematic, of course, is to substitute new forms and procedures for traditional materials, especially in large systems. It's possible, however, to create a compromise; to insert material focused on families into mandatory practices. As an example, family-oriented "prompts" have been developed for case managers who are interviewing an applicant for mental health services. Though all case managers working in the system must complete a standard statewide form, the form has been elaborated by staff and administrators interested in maintaining a family orientation. The information obtained through the additional prompts allows for a fuller understanding of the client's family situation and a more inclusive involvement of family members in the planning of services. Such adaptations are most readily managed by personnel within the system, but they can also be initiated as suggestions by outside personnel. Whatever the source, modifications of this kind sustain the family orientation of the workers as they proceed through the mandatory routines of their work.

The third factor, *an ability to recognize and connect system elements*, reflects our theoretical point of view and may require some explanation. When professional staff meet with a new client, we believe they should be prepared to work with two systems: the family network of the client and the various agencies that will be delivering services. Official papers don't highlight systemic connections, but we consider this perspective essential for understanding a situation and working effectively.

There's an interesting difference between family systems and organizational systems. Members of the client's family are in constant interaction, and if one meets with them, it's possible to see how they function. Agencies in the organizational network, however, are not usually in contact. Each subsystem in a case delivers services within its specialty—housing, judicial decisions, drug programs, foster care, or counseling—and, as we have pointed out at many points, the messages and mandates may be at cross-purposes.

What's required of the worker in relation to a client is to bring the family together, using knowledge and skill to understand the established patterns of this system and to help its members explore constructive ways of relating. What's required in relation to agency services is to create actual connections between subsystems that usually function separately—initiating contacts, encouraging communication, and facilitating conflict resolution. Those tasks require that workers should become alert to family patterns and skillful in bringing together parts of a system that control different services. Once established, that mind-set and the associated skills can become available to the staff during the training and in subsequent years.

The preparation of professionals to recognize and work with family systems has been thoroughly discussed throughout the chapters. We've said less, however, about encouraging alertness to connections at the level of organizations, or about how to bring subsystems together. We've taught these aspects in two ways: by creating structures in the training that model the connections among separate elements, and by outreach on the part of consultants and trainers that bring representatives of different subsystems into discussion.

Perhaps the most obvious example of structures that illustrate subsystem connections comes from the foster care project. Foster parents and agency workers were trained together as a team, since that's the way they should be working in the agency, and foster parents, birth parents, and caseworkers were brought together in a collaborative network to share information and solve problems on behalf of the child. An additional example is the use of two-person teams to work with a group throughout their training. With two trainers on the scene, they're able to serve different functions during the training sessions, but they also offer a model of how different points of view can be expressed and can move heated discussions toward a constructive resolution—a situation likely to arise and need handling when different corners of the helping establishment are brought together.

In some situations, the composition of the training groups exemplified subsystem collaboration, especially when the participants were part of a large service system. In the mental health project, for example, trainees came from different agencies and meetings rotated among their home sites. As a result, participants gained a broader understanding of how different agencies interpreted similar tasks, organized their operations, and integrated a family orientation into the way they functioned.

Outreach that brings together providers from separate agencies is generally initiated by consultants or trainers. They may also create collaborative groups within an agency, and these groups may continue to meet independently. Multidisciplinary case conferences in a large public hospital, for example, were originally convened by the project consultant, who brought together personnel from different departments who were working with the same clients. Once established, these conferences became a regular feature, attracting additional personnel from the hospital who were interested in the process.

More often, the process of connecting parts of a system centers on a particular situation and arises because there is a specific problem: Representatives of a drug treatment center and a foster care agency are brought together, for instance, because their conflicting demands are confusing and depressing the client; or the decision-making power of a hospital administrator is invoked in order to resolve staff disagreements about the presence of babies with positive toxicity on the wards; or a consultant contacts (or urges personnel to contact) influential figures in the hierarchy of the system in order to explore a particular issue with lawyers, judges, physicians, or agency administrators whose limited information is blocking the decisions of professionals with less power.

Such active attempts to integrate parts of a system are not always successful, but they are always worth the effort. At the least, they introduce a new idea to people brought into the situation; at the same time, they offer a model for workers who will continue in these settings, reinforcing the basic point that parts of a service system are connected and interactive, whether knowingly or not, and suggesting that it is a worker's task to encourage contact and communication.

CONSISTENT FAMILY-ORIENTED PROCEDURES WITHIN THE ORGANIZATION

Even well-trained, confident practitioners require the support of an organizational framework that has absorbed family-oriented practices into the ongoing work. The process of creating such a situation depends on the commitment and efforts of institutional leaders, the mobilization and involvement of staff and recipients as stakeholders, and the exercise of adaptability as required by the particular setting. If an institution maintains a consistent framework for working with clients, supervising staff, and informing new workers that "this is the way we do things," the orientation is stable and is likely to endure.

At the end of our training projects, as we have described them in earlier chapters, only the residence for substance-dependent adolescents, a relatively small and privately run institution, had developed a *pervasive family-oriented framework* for its activities. In the several situations where the system was large and complex, the effects were generally partial, primarily affecting a geographical area within a state, certain departments within an institution, or some agencies within the system. We view that result with a mixture of concern and optimism. Efforts to create change have been going on, with mixed results, from the beginning of time, and we take some comfort from a piece of wisdom written more than a century ago (and forgivable for its purely male perspective because of the time period): ". . . men fight and lose the battle, and the thing that they fought for comes about in spite of their defeat, and when it comes turns out not to be what they meant, and other men have to fight for what they meant under another name" (Morris, 1888). What we concentrate on, therefore, is the fact that changes *have* been integrated into the daily work of some service organizations as a result of the interventions, and more are likely to come about over time.

We have noted already that *family-oriented tools and procedures* organize the work of the staff and solidify the development of skillful practitioners. They also contribute to the survival of a family orientation within the setting. When such materials are created and become part of the daily routine, they convey a constant message about what the institution considers important and how things should be done. Beyond such operational procedures, however, the integration of a family perspective into an ongoing system depends on the attitudes and activities of the people involved—administrators, staff, and the recipients of service, as well as the consultants and trainers who bring new ideas into the system.

The *commitment of leaders* is crucial to this integration. In a sense, consultants and trainers are the driving force behind change; they must be persistent and creative if their ideas are to take effect. But it is the commitment of administrators and supervisors within the system that determines whether a new way of working will become integrated into the organization.

Wherever our interventions have had an effect, the work has been facilitated by personnel at executive and supervisory levels. They handled the necessities of space, time, and staff coverage, and used their contacts and influence to mobilize people and implement decisions. Their encouragement of the staff during the training smoothed the process, and they facilitated the structures and activities that continued to support the learning after the trainers had departed.

Commitment of this kind depends basically on personal style and, perhaps, on a professional perspective that is in agreement with the framework of the intervention. For people in leadership positions, however, there are always competing demands, and even willing collaborators are more likely to respond actively if the proponents of a new program keep contact, convey their recognition of administrative efforts, and provide periodic feedback.

The *mobilization and involvement of stakeholders* emerged as a relevant factor, and it applied both to institutional staff and to the recipients of service. As a matter of course, consultants and trainers expected that if the training was effective, administrators and workers would become stakeholders in a family-oriented approach, convinced of its value and concerned with maintaining family-based practices. It was surprising, however, that the intervention also affected the attitudes of the people receiving services. As they were drawn into family activities, some recipients became active participants, capable of influencing the continuation of such activities in the organizations that served them.

The clearest example of such a development came from the substance abuse programs. The people we have labeled as stakeholders in those two projects had quite different characteristics—pregnant and poor substance-dependent women in one group, parents of substance-dependent adolescents in the other. The differences between the two groups made three things clear: *first*, that whatever their life situations, most people seeking help expect to have little say concerning the kind of service they receive, either because their social status and past experiences have made them passive or because they do not feel equipped to challenge the procedures and decisions of a professional staff; *second*, that the stakeholders in a situation may be either the actual recipients of service, as in the case of the pregnant women, or interested family members, such as parents in cases where the client is a child; and, *third*, that the task of mobilizing people and helping them to become active stakeholders requires motivation and skill on the part of professional staff.

In both situations, clients and their families needed to be drawn into family-oriented activities—such as discussion groups, family sessions, family associations—and they began as passive participants, with consultants or staff members as their leaders. With time and accumulated experience, however, they developed their own leaders and created activities that reached out to newcomers and the community. At that point, they were involved in a family approach, and had become stakeholders in the maintenance of family-oriented patterns in their service settings.

Though we did not mobilize family-oriented stakeholders in

other projects, the possibility is worth exploring in almost any setting. Fraenkel (2006) has developed a collaborative program with the stakeholders in homeless families, and groups concerned with the rights and roles of families have appeared spontaneously in the area of mental health. The latter have sometimes made professional people uneasy, since they are seen as advocates and potential adversaries. It seems useful, however, to establish common cause with clients and families who wish to be included in planning and treatment, and to negotiate agreements between professionals and stakeholders, as necessary, concerning boundaries and roles. If they are admitted into the healing and service process, stakeholders often have a natural understanding of the relevance of the family network and will serve as a factor in preserving this systemic way of organizing services.

Adaptability is both an attitude and a way of functioning. Without reasonable flexibility in presenting new ideas and adapting to changing circumstances, a new approach probably cannot be integrated into an established system or survive over time. This may be particularly true with regard to the large public service systems, where there are constant shifts in policies and personnel.

As we moved from one project to another, our basic views never varied; we always believed that service must be provided for the individual in the context of the family, and that both families and agencies must be understood as interactive systems. But we made many adaptations to the conditions of different settings, to the background and preparation of different training groups, and to the problems and life circumstances of the people who came for help. We needed to pick our issues carefully when we dealt with the staff of the therapeutic drug treatment community, letting some important aspects go, but could help the substance-dependent women work on meaningful family problems in their discussion groups. We needed to accept mandatory forms that were oriented toward individual pathology, in large systems, but could demonstrate the relevance of family and the nature of their strengths in family sessions. We had little effect on the dominance of psychiatric diagnoses or the prevalence of heavy medication, in particular settings, but could help a staff understand that the suicidal impulses of an adolescent were interwoven with the impact of immigration and minority status on the way her family functioned. Bringing a family-oriented approach into such settings requires a constant adaptation to what is possible, as well as a reformulation as necessary of how to teach, work with clients, and affect how things are done.

To state that adaptability is a factor that facilitates the survival of a particular approach runs contrary to views that have become prevalent in the professional field; that is, the current emphasis on clearly specified methods that should be put into practice without deviation, and the preference for evidence-based procedures that have been assessed through tightly designed studies measuring specific results. It's our contention that those criteria cannot be met in working with complicated families, except by limiting the conditions and the goals, and that they do not apply well to work in the public sector, where changing realities require creative adaptations. Professionals who work in those situations need to function flexibly within a stable framework of ideas, and must decide what aspects of their method they can give up, when the circumstances demand it, without sacrificing the basic premises of their approach.

The discrepancy between the view that a new approach will not become part of an institution unless it has flexible features and the more prevalent view that interventions should be researched and carefully controlled is actually part of a larger issue concerning the social and ideological tenor of the times.

SOCIAL SUPPORT FOR FAMILY-ORIENTED PRACTICES

Here we are concerned with the prevailing social climate of the culture—an umbrella category affecting all efforts to help people who depend on public services. Sometimes, *social policies* are benign with respect to underprivileged populations; at other times, they offer little encouragement for the procedures we have been proposing. To gain perspective and think realistically, it's necessary to look at history, and to consider both the social and professional matters that have affected the provision of services to poor and needy people.

We can start with a gauntlet thrown down by Don Jackson, a systems-oriented psychiatrist writing 50 years ago, who argued that the individual does not exist. The concept, he maintained, was an intellectual construction, achieved by erasing the social connections among people (Jackson, 1957). His statement was a political act, a broadside against the ideology of individual psychodynamics, but it was also a moral statement about human existence. The credo of family therapy was that individuals *are* in relationships—that is, that existence is defined by connections.

A decade or so later, when we began working with welfare families and the social agencies that regulate their lives, we were also entering a political arena. We had taken on the task of offering psychologically sophisticated services to people who were often considered hard or impossible to reach. In so doing, we were supporting the right of the welfare population to relevant services, and we were engaging ourselves in the search for ways of formulating those services so they would be meaningful and helpful for this population.

In retrospect, it's clear that we were aided by the ethos of those times. Johnson's War on Poverty had been proclaimed, Black was Beautiful, and social issues were at the forefront of national concern. Energy and funding were available for creative projects that would reach needy populations. Governmental and private foundations supported our initial work with families and delinquent children, as well as our project to develop indigenous family counselors who would work in the community. As time went on, the climate—social, political, economic—continued to encourage exploration and innovation in working with poor families and with the agencies that served them.

Now, in the new millennium, the War on Poverty has been replaced by the War on Terrorism. Given the emphasis on protection and survival, poverty has moved to the periphery of the political consciousness. The immediate result, in a time of high budget deficits, is a decrease in services available for the poor. Specific effects include the development of more stringent requirements for assistance with food, shelter, and child support, and extend as well to services that have to do with health, family relationships, and psychological well-being. In this atmosphere, it has become more difficult to pursue and implement our work.

Oddly enough, current scientific advances have had some of the same limiting effects. Neurological research, for example, has pinpointed areas in the brain that control affect and mood disorders. Although fascinating in themselves, discoveries of this nature have threatened the conceptual advances that came somewhat earlier, including the increase in our knowledge of how systems function and can be changed.

The new scientific information has had repercussions throughout the corporate world and the psychological professions. At least for the present, the emphasis is on creating specific remedies for particular ailments and on documenting their success in relieving symptoms. The chemical industry has provided "silver bullets" for specific diagnoses, and psychiatry has increased its reliance on medication to control psychological symptoms. The profession provides less training in psychotherapy for its young practitioners than it formerly did, as well as less preparation for understanding the complex social networks within which the suffering of their patients is expressed. Even family therapists have become competitive in the search for certainty, organizing their work so it can provide evidence of the effectiveness of their interventions. To an extent, of course, these trends are an adaptation to the perspective of the HMOs, which connect diagnoses to specific treatments and reimburse accordingly.

None of us would interfere with the continuous flow of new scientific information or ignore the palliative effects of medication on depression, confusion, or other painful states of mind. Nor would we question the value of evaluating the effects of our work. But new information should enhance, rather than replace, previous advances. We should not push aside the explorations of experienced and skillful practitioners who work with families in favor of a medical cocktail for each family member. We should not automatically applaud the strict adherence to treatment manuals meant to ensure identical interventions by all therapists. And we should not expect pills to help a poverty-stricken, drug-dependent single mother deal effectively with her reality. The advances in knowledge should be integrated with an understanding that life is complex, that relationships are formative and essential, and that the relief that comes from immediate remedies will generally require a second stage of intervention, in which attention is paid to the context of the individual and a variety of professional skills are required.

We have devoted this book to describing that framework and those skills, and to considering how constructive changes in the service systems can be made to last over time. The introduction of procedures that include families in treatment and emphasize the coordination of services involves swimming against the current in times such as these, and that is always difficult. It requires tenacity, endurance, and a concern for the human suffering of people at the bottom rung of society. It also requires a degree of optimism. We know, via history and experience, that times change. Especially with social support, but even without it, the teaching of new ideas can take effect; institutions can integrate more constructive ways of working; and professionals can become broader, more compassionate, and more effective in their contact with individuals and families. We hope that readers will be part of such changes, and that they will experience their efforts as worthwhile.

References

Burns, B. J., & Goldman, S. K. (1998). *Promising practices in wrap-around for children with severe emotional disturbance and their families.* In Center for Mental Health Services, *Systems of care: Promising practices in children's mental health.* Rockville, MD: Center for Mental Health Services, Substance Abuse and Mental Health Administration, U.S. Department of Health and Human Services.

Colapinto, J. (1995). Dilution of family process in social services: Implications for treatment of neglectful families. *Family Process, 34,* 59–74.

DeMuro, P., & Rideout, P. (2002). *Team decision-making: Involving the family and community in child welfare decisions.* Baltimore: Annie E. Casey Foundation.

Egelko, S., Galanter, M., Dermatis, H., & DeMaio, C. (1998). Evaluation of a multi-systems model for treating perinatal cocaine addiction. *Journal of Substance Abuse Treatment, 15,* 251–259.

Fraenkel, P. (2006). Engaging families as experts: Collaborative family program development. *Family Process, 45,* 237–257.

Grimes, K. E. (2003). Collaboration with primary care: Sharing risks, goals and outcomes in an integrated system of care. In A. J. Pumariega & N. C. Winters (Eds.), *The handbook of child and adolescent systems of care: The new community psychiatry.* San Francisco: Jossey-Bass.

Haley, J. (1976). *Problem-solving therapy.* New York: Harper & Row.

Henggeler, S. W., Schoenwald, S. K., Borduin, C. M., Rowland, M. D., & Cunningham, P. B. (1998). *Multisystemic treatment of antisocial behavior in children and adolescents.* New York: Guilford Press.

Jackson, D. (1957). The question of family homeostasis. *Psychiatric Quarterly Supplement, 31,* 79–90.

Liddle, H. A. (2002). *Multidimensional family therapy treatment (MDFT) for adolescent cannabis users.* Rockville, MD: Substance Abuse and Mental Health Services Administration.

Liddle, H. A., & Rowe, C. L. (Eds.). (2006). *Adolescent substance abuse: Research and clinical advances.* Cambridge, UK: Cambridge University Press.

Marx, L., Benoit, M., & Kamradt, B. (2003). Foster children in the child welfare system. In A. J. Pumariega & N. C. Winters (Eds.), *The handbook of child and adolescent systems of care: The new community psychiatry.* San Francisco: Jossey-Bass.

McDaniel, S., Campbell, T., & Seaburn, D. (1995). Principles for collaboration between health and mental health providers in primary care. *Family Systems Medicine, 13,* 283–298.

Miller, S. M., McDaniel, S. H., Rolland, J., & Feetham, S. (Eds.). (2006). *Individuals, families, and the new era of genetics: Biopsychosocial perspectives.* New York: Norton.

Minuchin, P. (1995). Foster and natural families: Forming a cooperative network. In L. Combrinck-Graham (Ed.), *Children in families at risk.* New York: Guilford Press.

Minuchin, P., with Brooks, A., Colapinto, J., Genijovich, E., Minuchin, D., & Minuchin, S. (1990). *Training manual for foster parents.* New York: Family Studies, Inc. (Available from National Resource Center for Family Centered Practice, 100 Oakdale Campus, Room W206OH, Iowa City, IA, 52242-5000).

Minuchin, S. (1984). *Family kaleidoscope.* Cambridge, MA: Harvard University Press.

Minuchin, S., Nichols, M., & Lee, W. (2007). *Assessing families and couples: From symptom to system.* Boston: Allyn & Bacon.

Morris, W. (1888). *A Dream of John Ball.* (Available at *ebooks@Adelaide* 2004).

Nichols, M. P., & Schwartz, R. C. (Eds.). (2004). *Family therapy: Concepts and methods* (6th ed.). Boston: Allyn & Bacon.

Pumariega, A. J., & Winters, N. C. (Eds.). (2003). *The handbook of child and adolescent systems of care: The new community psychiatry.* San Francisco: Jossey-Bass.

Rowe, C. L., & Liddle, H. A. (2003). Substance abuse. *Journal of Marital and Family Therapy, 29,* 97–120.

Sharkey, M. (1997). *Family to family: Bridging families, communities and child welfare.* Baltimore: Annie E. Casey Foundation.

Stanton, D. M., & Heath, A. S. (2004). Family/couples approaches to treatment engagement and therapy. In J. H. Lowinson, P. Ruiz, R. B. Millman, & J. G. Langrod (Eds.), *Substance abuse: A comprehensive textbook* (4th ed.). Baltimore: Lippincott Williams & Wilkins.

Stroul, B. A. (2003). Systems of care: A framework for children's mental health care. In A. J. Pumariega & N. C. Winters (Eds.), *The handbook of child and adolescent systems of care: The new community psychiatry.* San Francisco: Jossey-Bass.

Szapocznik, J., Hervis, O. E., & Schwartz, S. (2003). *Brief Strategic Family Therapy for adolescent drug abuse* (NIH Publication No. 03-4751). Rockville, MD: National Institute on Drug Abuse.

Thielman, B. (2001). *Implementing the values and strategies of family to family.* Baltimore: Annie E. Casey Foundation.

VanDenBerg, J. & Grealish, E. (1996). Individualized services and supports through the wraparound process: Philosophy and procedures. *Journal of Child and Family Studies, 5,* 7–21.

Index